P9-CAE-974

Bha

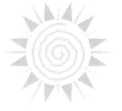

The

POWER CONSCIOUS BREATHING

DATE DUE

AUG 1 8 1999	
SEP 1 8 1999	
OCT 0 9 1999	
FEB 0 8 2003	
9-15-03 ILL	
JAN 0 3 2005	
MAR 2 9 2005	
OCT 1 7 2005	
AUG 0 7 2006	
MAY 1 8 2009	
AUG 1 6 2011	
DEC 0 8 2015	

BRODART, CO.   Cat. No. 23-221-003

Stamps noted 5-9-11

VASANTHI BHAT

i

First published in 1997 by
Vasanthi Bhat
1196 Lynbrook Way
San Jose, CA 95129

© Vasanthi Bhat 1997
All rights reserved. This book is protected under the copyright laws of the United States of America and other countries. No part of this book may be copied, photocopied, or reproduced in any manner without the written consent of the author.

Credits:
Published by Vasanthi Bhat
Edited by: Rich Slogar
Photography: Mahabaleshwar K.P. Bhat
Book and Cover Design: Amita Shenoi

ISBN #0-9655499-0-9

Printed in the United States of America by:
Bertelsmann Industry Services, Inc.

This book is

dedicated to my

Parents

When my father passed away all I could think of was his simple and generous life-style. He lived a quiet, humble life with deep compassion for the poor and needy. He helped thousands of underprivileged and less fortunate people during the course of his life. But even with a simple and compassionate life-style, he always seemed to be under stress. He passed away due to an ulcer which developed into cancer. I wish I had an opportunity to teach him yoga to help relieve his stress. But at that time, I was still learning and experimenting with yoga in my own life. However, using his life's example, I vowed to carry on his work in my own way.

As for my mother, her most admirable quality was that she never compared her children to anyone. She simply accepted us for who we were. She never criticized anyone; instead, she would encourage us with kind and gentle advice. I am glad that I had an opportunity to teach my mother some yoga techniques that gave her relief from her arthritic condition in the latter years of her life.

I am very grateful to have had parents who possessed unique and invaluable qualities which directly helped and influenced me through every stage of my life.

CONTENTS

CONTENTS

About Vasanthi Bhat

Vasanthi was born and raised in India. Since childhood, she has shown great enthusiasm and interest in a variety of sports. She participated in many athletic activities and won several awards. She also participated in a variety of fine arts, such as singing and dancing. Vasanthi was married in 1971 and subsequently moved to Canada in 1972.

She began practicing Richard Hittleman's yoga in Canada in 1975 to relieve her migraine headaches, reduce anxiety, and gain control of her weight after having two children. After only a few sessions, she began to feel better. Gradually, these symptoms left her and she gained the ability to balance her physical and mental energy, which led to a greater sense of inner peace. As a result, she fell in love with yoga for it showed her the path to her inner self through stretching, breathing, and meditation. This experience inspired her to seek more intensive training at the Bihar School of Yoga in Bangalore, India under Swami Satyananda Saraswati. For spiritual fulfillment, she also adopted the teachings of her teacher's guru Swami Sivananda.

Over the years, people who knew Vasanthi started noticing some remarkable changes in her and the positive effects yoga had on her life. They asked her to teach them yoga. In 1976, she began teaching and giving demonstrations at various clubs and organizations in Bangalore, India. After years of practicing and teaching yoga, Vasanthi realized that stress was the root cause of all ailments. Stress causes the body to reduce the flow of vital energy or prana to the various parts of the body. Proper breathing and stretching techniques can improve the circulation of prana and help heal many ailments. To share this knowledge with others, she developed a unique and gentle, yet powerful teaching style for people of all ages and all physical conditions.

In 1985, Vasanthi moved to California and has been teaching under the name Vasantha Yoga for Health and Fitness. In June 1989, Vasanthi started teaching yoga at colleges and several major US corporations such as Intel, Quantum, LSI Logic, Northern Telecom, and Sun Microsystems. She currently teaches at De Anza College and companies such as Sensys Instruments, Cisco Systems, Exodus, and Novartis Crop Protection, Inc. She also teaches private groups for students of all ages and different levels. In addition, she also volunteers her time giving yoga classes at community centers for seniors where she incorporates Dr. Ramesh Kapadia's universal healing techniques for reversing heart disease, preventing various ailments, and maintaining general health. She also presents lectures and demonstrations, and holds workshops at various institutions. To date, she has taught yoga to over 10,000 people, ranging in age from 5 to 95.

She also conducts teachers' training programs for her advanced students to enable them to teach at various corporate facilities, health clubs, and senior centers.

Vasanthi released her first instructional yoga video in June 1993. In June 1994, she released six more videos and an audio tape for all age groups. Another set of six new yoga videos and a compact disk on meditation were released in September 1996. Her products are appreciated in the United States and around the world.

Vasanthi's specialty is teaching people how to combine asanas (postures), pranayama (breathing), and meditation so students can achieve maximum healing and a sense of well-being. Her gentle hatha yoga teaching style encourages students to work at their own pace and to adopt yoga as a vital and integral part of their lives.

At the time of this publication, Vasanthi has been married for 26 years and has a 24-year old daughter and a 22-year old son. In her spare time, Vasanthi enjoys gardening and brisk walks. She is fond of eastern as well as western dance and music. She is also a great believer in the holistic approach to healing. Her role as parent, teacher, writer, producer, distributor, and homemaker are very demanding; yet her secret to achieving her goals is simple and available to everyone — **regular yoga practice and conscious breathing**!

A Few Words to My Readers

My dream is to let people know that conscious breathing and yoga are basically very simple, yet profoundly powerful healing skills that can be practiced by anyone. Whenever I was in public places, I observed the breathing habits of people around me. To my surprise, I noticed that what the yogis said was so true — most people do not breathe properly. This motivated me to write this book to help people adopt conscious breathing techniques in their lives.

This book is specifically written to help people of all ages and all physical conditions (including the handicapped) realize the value of conscious breathing during postures, meditation, and daily activities. The techniques I describe are versatile and can be utilized at your convenience to alleviate stress, stress-related ailments, and mental barriers. In turn, you will regain your vital energy and experience physical and mental equilibrium and good health. This vital energy will expand your potential and help you achieve inner peace for a healthy, happy, and productive life.

Based on my teaching experience and feedback from thousands of students who have benefited and are still benefiting, I assure you that positive results can be achieved if you practice the described techniques with an open mind and patient acceptance.

Please keep in mind not to strain yourself at any time when practicing these techniques. Listen to your body when you practice stretching and breathing. You may begin your practice at any level from basic to advanced, since flexibility is not a prerequisite to practice yoga. Remember not to use force to perform advanced techniques. Even in the simplest postures, you can achieve noticeable results if you remember to relax and stretch correctly while breathing consciously. Understand that it is very dangerous for the heart and the entire system to practice these techniques without proper breath control. In addition, make sure to check with your physician before starting this or any exercise program.

Remember, everyone possesses a power within. As you practice these techniques, you will notice that power coming forth, allowing you to control and utilize your vital force or prana in your daily life. The personal power you regain is profound and wonderful beyond any other power in the world. It is beautiful and precious. Most importantly, it can be shared with others, but it can never be taken away from you.

Vasanthi

Acknowledgments

I am infinitely grateful to the Supreme Power for guiding me through every stage of my life—especially in my practice of yoga. I have always received the proper inspiration to do the right things for myself as well as for others.

My respects to **Richard Hittleman**, **Swami Satyananda Saraswati**, **Swami Sivananda**, and **Swami Satchidananda** for imparting their gentle and easy-to-learn techniques.

I began learning yogic postures from Richard Hittleman. His teachings relieved my headaches, toned my muscles, and contributed to my weight loss. My sense of well-being was heightened by the fact that I started looking and feeling youthful again.

Swami Satyananda Saraswati, my guru, helped me learn many techniques to purify myself and achieve inner harmony.

Through the teachings that Swami Sivananda passed on to my guru, I learned the philosophy of "working hard to purify" in order to achieve a balance in life.

By viewing Swami Satchidananda's videos and reading his articles, I have indirectly learned many additional techniques and skills, especially simplicity.

All my students have also contributed to the development of my classes and this book. Their intense motivation to continue learning for many years, inspired me to continue teaching. I thank and respect all my students for their encouragement and support. A special thanks to my students who shared their personal experiences in this book.

Publishing this book was no small task as it involved tremendous dedication and sacrifice on my part as well as those associated with the book. In this regard I wish to express my endless gratitude to the following people. Thanks to Amita Shenoi, a graphic designer, who designed the entire book and assisted with the final editing process. My thanks to Rich Slogar, a technical writer, for editing the book from early drafts to the final version and providing valuable suggestions in the design process in spite of his busy work schedule. I value Mr. Prakash Chandra Gupta, a retired additional general manager, Indian Railways, for his timely assistance in the final copy edit phase of the book. I appreciate Krishna Bhat's timely help with the final edits. I am very grateful to Jean Livingston for her timely support with partial edits. From Anjali Puri, a technical writer, I learned what it takes to write a book. Since this is my first book, her advice is greatly appreciated. Veena Bhat, my daughter, and Supriya Bhat, my niece, assisted in editing and most importantly helped me express some of my true feelings about yoga. Most of the asanas I have demonstrated in the pages to follow were photographed by my husband Mahabaleshwar Bhat, an engineer by profession. Some photographs were contributed by my nephew, Kumaraswamy, a professional videographer. I thank Kokila Patel, a registered physical therapist, for her professional advice and views on yoga's relevance in her field. I also appreciate the valuable expert opinions from Mala Seshagiri, a dietician, on the subject of nutrition.

Finally, I wish to express that if it were not for my husband and childrens' sensitivity to my needs and their ongoing support, understanding, and encouragement, I could not have published this book while conducting my numerous classes and producing my yoga videos. My mother-in-law, Saraswathi Amma, not only encouraged me but also provided domestic support when I needed it most.

San Jose, California   **Vasanthi**

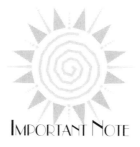

Important Note

Never force or strain your body when attempting the techniques described and recommended in this book or products listed herein. Consult your physician before attempting any poses. The author/publisher disclaims any implied warranties or merchantability of liability, loss, or injury in connection with any of these techniques and products.

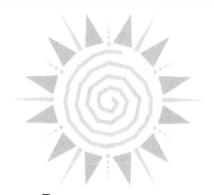

INTRODUCING
THE POWER OF CONSCIOUS BREATHING

"Controlled conscious breathing is a natural tranquilizer
and a powerful healer."

All of us work hard in life to accomplish our personal goals. Sometimes, we work so hard that we forget the vital force within us; we breathe automatically, not taking the time to breathe consciously. The daily automatic breathing controlled by our involuntary systems merely sustains our lives, not using our lungs to their fullest capacity. Starved of oxygen, we let our health and stress-related problems intensify, creating a vicious cycle of stress, tension, and oxygen deprivation. As days, months, and years pass, our bodies show signs of wear or sickness, and our emotions become unsteady or compulsive. These are signs that prana (the wonderful, free, healing energy) needs to be consciously directed throughout the body.

Prana is the vital air or energy. **Yama** is the control or direction of that vital energy. Pranayama is the control and direction of vital life energy through conscious breathing. During pranayama, breathing becomes the center of our awareness. The mind focuses solely on the breath. We consciously observe and control the amount, length, and retention of our breath. Our breathing becomes voluntary, specific, and regulated. The enhanced breathing of pranayama oxygenates the blood and allows healing energy to flow through the circulation of the life fluids to all parts of the body. As a result, the body becomes revitalized and rejuvenated by this enriched supply of life's vital force. With the continued practice of pranayama, we can even learn to quiet and control our minds. Eventually, we can learn to direct the vital energy to other aspects of our lives through breathing and visualization. We can learn to reduce stress, heal specific ailments, and develop deeper concentration to achieve inner peace.

The ancient yogis predicted thousands of years ago that no matter how much the world advances in technological development, when it comes to the aspect of health, we will have to put aside the technical innovations and relearn the ancient yogic techniques in order to relax the body and mind. Unless we take the time to relax and understand what is happening within the body and mind, there will be no cure for our stress-related health problems.

The origin of pranayama (conscious breathing) is in hatha yoga — the practice of combining postures (asanas), conscious breathing (pranayama), and meditation. The postures of hatha yoga date back more than 5,000 years to pre-Vedic times. Among the archaeological excavations of Harappa and Mohenjadaro, India, where people of pre-Aryan civilization lived, statues were found demonstrating yogic poses. The ancient yogis also observed animals in nature and adopted aspects from their naturally healthy behavior and breathing patterns. By observing and imitating the different postures of the animals, the yogis were able to live longer and healthier lives. The humming of the bee (brahmari) and the lion's breath (simha's breath) are a few of breathing techniques the yogis derived from the animals. Through the turtle pose, which relaxes the body as can be seen from the resting position of the turtle, they learned how to retain energy. From the locust pose, they were able to release energy from the base of the spine, as does the grasshopper in its stretching position.

It is said that originally there were thousands of asanas. Over the course of centuries, these asanas were modified and reduced by experienced yogis to a few hundred. Out of these few hundred asanas, about 30-50 remain in modern day practice. Similarly, there were hundreds of pranayama techniques, of which only about 15-30 techniques are generally practiced.

Eventually, hatha yoga[1] became an integral part of the eightfold yogic path to healing and enlightenment. These eight yogic paths are:

1. **Yama:** non-violence
2. **Niyama:** discipline and cleanliness, both external and internal
3. **Asana:** postures
4. **Pranayama:** controlled or conscious breathing
5. **Pratyahara:** controlling the senses
6. **Dharana:** concentration
7. **Dhyana:** meditation
8. **Samadhi:** inner peace and higher consciousness

These eight paths can be practiced separately or together in combination. When practiced together, they complement each other and lead to the achievement of the highest physical and spiritual level. When combining the paths, the hatha yoga sequence of asanas (3rd path), pranayama (4th path), and meditation (7th path) works best and naturally leads to the attainment of the other paths. Conscious breathing in the asanas helps relax the body and direct prana to the appropriate parts. This has the ability to control the senses (5th path). Conscious breathing in the asanas also strengthens the pranic channels and prepares the body for the practice of pranayama. Regular practice of pranayama circulates prana throughout the body and mind. The circulation of prana helps improve concentration (6th path), develop discipline (2nd path), heal ailments, and revitalize the mind and body. This revitalization of the mind and body naturally opens the pathway to meditation (7th path). Meditation expands consciousness by promoting inner peace (8th path), which elevates the soul to practice non-violence (1st path). It is conscious breathing throughout the sequence of asanas, pranayama, and meditation that leads the practitioner from one path to the other.

[1] There are also other forms of yoga that are practiced to attain enlightenment, such as bhakti yoga (devotion), gnana yoga (knowledge), and karma yoga (action).

Pranayama, the control of vital energy through conscious breathing, is the most essential path in all the yogic paths and the foundation to achieve all other paths.

Pranayama can be practiced by people of all ages and all physical conditions. In addition, these breathing techniques are very portable and do not require any special equipment other than your own body. They can even be done quietly without anyone needing to know what you are doing. Unlike aerobics and other exercises, pranayama takes a minimal amount of energy, and therefore, even the sick or aged can practice it. Pranayama oxygenates the blood, balances the endocrine system, and relaxes the entire system.

Conscious breathing (pranayama) helps us gain control over our daily situations. One simple example is to monitor your breathing when under stress. The stress may come from either an external or internal source, but it manifests itself in the body in similar ways. Usually, stress elevates the heart rate, increases rapid or shallow breathing, and distracts the mind. The symptoms of tension, headaches, muscle aches, nervousness, and anxiety arise due to improper breathing during stressful times. If we consciously breathe slowly, we will be able to relax the mind, which will help us find positive solutions to stressful situations. Our breathing affects our thinking, and our thinking affects our breath. Whenever a stressful situation occurs, remember to either breathe slowly to gain control over the mind or think positively in order to relax the breath. Unless we take the time to relax and discern what is happening within the body and mind, other techniques will not solve our stress-related health problems. Therefore, regular practice of conscious breathing is important. It takes strong discipline to develop conscious breathing since we normally rely on an involuntary breathing system.

There is a danger for people who practice asanas or meditation without controlled breathing. This type of practice should be done with great caution! Breathing incorrectly while practicing postures strains the body. Unless we learn how to breathe steadily, we will find it difficult to meditate due to the lack of concentration. This strain and lack of concentration will lead to the development of anxiety, headaches, hypertension, and finally stress, due to the lack of oxygen in the body. Additional pain and discomfort may follow. Conversely, when steady breathing is consciously practiced during asanas and meditation, the body receives the maximum benefit, and the mind naturally experiences a peaceful, meditative state. Conscious breathing is the key to experiencing happiness, contentment, and inner peace.

Helen Keller is known to have said, "The best and most beautiful things in the world cannot be seen or even touched, they must be felt with the heart." If we put aside the modern struggle for finding fulfillment from outside of ourselves and practice conscious breathing, we can learn to access our inner wisdom to relieve stress, improve health, and experience happiness.

I practice asanas to relieve accumulated tension, improve circulation, and maintain health. I also practice pranayama and meditation to assist in balancing my emotions and energy. Whenever an unpredictable or difficult situation occurs, just 2-3 rounds of alternate nostril breathing or deep breathing restores my emotional balance. In addition to these benefits, it enables me to increase my awareness throughout the day to expand my spirituality.

The following examples of my students' experiences show that everyone, regardless of age and physical condition, can benefit from hatha yoga techniques.

Registered nurse relieves colds and other ailments

To benefit her health Jane Berto, a registered nurse, says, "I do the alternate nostril breathing daily, and I have not had a cold since I joined Vasanthi's class seven years ago." She also started teaching hatha yoga to her patients to relax their neck, shoulders, and wrist joints, and promote their healing.

Eleven year old increases stamina

To eliminate stress and relax the mind, 11-year old Tanay Dudhela practices pranayama before running the mile. He maintains that it builds up his stamina and enables him to run longer without getting tired.

Woman eases birth process

To prepare and recover from childbirth, Hazuki Kataoka used both asanas and pranayama. She claims it controlled her emotions and back pain, and assisted towards easy child birth.

Computer users ease stress

Many of my students claim that at work, just stepping back from their computer for a moment and practicing a few minutes of pranayama refreshes and revitalizes them for the rest of the afternoon. For some, tension headaches decrease as a response to the increased revitalizing energy.

Regardless of age or physical condition, you are ready to begin learning the ancient yogic techniques for relieving stress and improving health. Chapter 1 of this book guides you through the process of preparing your body to experience prana through the practice of asanas (postures). Remember, steady, conscious breathing during the asanas relaxes the muscles and helps alleviate stress. Without conscious breathing, these positive effects will be greatly diminished. Chapter 2 introduces the techniques of pranayama. Pranayama techniques will help you focus your senses and send the pranic energy to where it is needed. This process revitalizes your body and tranquilizes the mind. Chapter 3 describes the practice of meditation. You will learn how to quiet the mind and guide it to inner peace. Chapter 4 discusses how these techniques can be practiced to reduce injury and increase the enjoyment of exercise and other daily activities. Chapter 5 describes how to use the techniques of asanas, pranayama, and meditation in the workplace.

You can practice the techniques of asana, pranayama, and meditation together or separately if you wish. Choose what is most comfortable for you. However, if you do practice all three, practice them in the order of asanas, pranayama, and meditation. Use these valuable techniques to relieve stress, relax and tone muscles, maintain and improve health, improve concentration, regain energy, lose or gain weight, look and feel younger, or simply feel great. They can also help relieve conditions such as back-pain, headaches, high and low blood pressure, insomnia, depression, lung and heart ailments, and many other health problems.

Parents caring for children can rejuvenate themselves and recover from fatigue. Children can improve memory and concentration. Older adults can improve their strength, alertness, and memory. Healthy, active people without health problems can benefit too. For example, athletes, dancers, and others can practice these techniques before an activity to improve concentration and performance, after an activity to restore energy, or between activities to build up stamina and prevent injuries. Busy professionals can take time during working hours, work breaks, or travelling to refresh and renew themselves.

FREQUENTLY ASKED QUESTIONS

What time of day is best to practice yoga?

Although practicing yoga around sunrise or sunset is ideal because the outdoor environment is calm and your stomach is likely to be empty, it is important to pick a convenient time when you can practice with a clear mind. Be flexible and discover the time that is best for you.

If you just can't seem to find enough time to complete a routine, simply practice one or two postures or breathing exercises. Even a small effort will add up over time.

It is best to practice yoga on an empty stomach. When the stomach is full, the mind loses its concentration, due to increased blood flow to the digestive process. The practice of yoga draws blood away from the digestive process and may cause indigestion and cramps. Wait for approximately 1/2 hour after a drink, 1 hour after a light snack, 2 hours after a regular meal, and 3 hours after a heavy meal before practicing intense yoga that involves compression of the abdominal area. For warm-up purposes, no waiting is necessary. You can practice both standing and sitting warm-ups anytime to refresh quickly.

How long do I need to practice yoga to receive the benefits?

It is best to practice yoga everyday or every other day, depending on your needs and abilities. When pressed for time, try to practice yoga for at least 5-10 minutes. To improve general health, practice yoga for about 20 minutes. To condition the body or help alleviate ailments, practice for 30-60 minutes.

Your routine can even be divided during the day. For example, practice a few postures in the morning after waking. Do standing stretches and pranayama during work breaks and whenever you feel stressed and wish to revitalize yourself. Then, in the evening, practice several additional postures. By listening to your needs and dividing your practice sessions throughout the day, you can easily adopt a routine that is most beneficial for your body, mind, and emotions.

Should I change my diet or become a vegetarian to practice yoga?

There is no requirement to follow a strict vegetarian diet or to avoid certain foods. Contrary to popular opinion, yogis did not say that one must become a vegetarian. However, they emphasized the importance of including high fiber foods like vegetables, fruits, lentils, and whole grains, and minimizing the intake of stimulants and dehydrants such as coffee and alcohol. Foods from the high fiber group are easy to digest, have plenty of nutrients, and cleanse the intestines naturally. After regular practice of yoga, many people have a tendency to adopt a vegetarian diet. Listen to your body's needs and eat appropriately.

Can I practice yoga if I am seeing a doctor or taking medication?

If you are seeing a doctor, continue to do so. Let your doctor know that you plan to practice yoga. Although it is not necessary, it helps to work with a doctor or practitioner who respects yoga. It is also helpful to consult your physician regularly for checkups and seek his/her advice when any injury or lasting discomfort occurs.

If you have high blood pressure, take special care when practicing the inverted poses and poses in which your head is resting on the floor. If you have low blood pressure, carefully observe your breathing during each pose. If you experience any dizziness, come out of the pose immediately.

If you have a sore muscle or injury, you can still practice yoga. However, practice very gently. Do not strain the sore or injured area. Conscious breathing and visualization can be used to accelerate the healing process.

Can I practice yoga if I am pregnant?

If you have been practicing yoga before the pregnancy, continue your regular routine until the third month. After the third month, practice easy postures and be sure to keep your legs apart during any forward bending asanas. Be careful not to compress the abdominal area.

If you are new to yoga, practice yoga only under the guidance of an experienced teacher.

Refer to the list of resources after the appendices, for information on my video 'Yoga for Pregnant Women'.

Can I be involved in other athletic activities in parallel with yoga?

Yes. In fact, yoga complements all types of activities including aerobics, walking, swimming, running, and many others. Yoga increases the energy level and helps stretch and tone the muscles. In addition, yoga can be practiced to warm up and cool down to help prevent injuries and increase flexibility.

Can I practice yoga to lose weight?

Yes. This is one of the most commonly asked questions. Many of my students have not only achieved weight loss after practicing yoga, but have successfully maintained their weight. As a matter of fact, I began practicing yoga when I was overweight, and I have been able to maintain my desired weight.

Do I need to be aware of my body type[2], such as vata, pitta, and kapha in order to practice yoga?

Knowing your body type definitely helps you to select foods that suit your body's constitution. The regular practice of asanas, pranayama, and meditation helps balance the vata, pitta, and kapha tendencies.

---

[2] For detailed information on these body types, refer to books on Ayurveda.

Consciously Breathing in The Asanas

"When it comes to relaxation, just trust your body, mind, and breath. There are no solutions to your stressful situations unless you are willing to travel within."

Yoga means the experience of oneness or union with our inner being (self). This union is the mind uniting with the body and the breath to attain a higher level of consciousness. Mind, body, and breath are interconnected. For example, if we are emotionally disturbed, the body often responds with a loss of appetite and/or indigestion. Likewise, if we develop muscular tension from working at a computer too long or from driving for an extended period of time, we also experience mental fatigue. The connection between mind, body, and breath is also noticeable during other stressful situations, like trying to rush somewhere on a tight schedule or hurrying to meet an approaching deadline. In response to the stress, the upper back and neck muscles get tense and breathing becomes shallow. The goal of yoga is to take time out during our everyday experience to create a perfect union of our physical, mental, emotional, and spiritual states to promote good health and inner peace.

Asanas are postures in which we remain steady and comfortable both physically and mentally while breathing consciously for a desired length of time without strain. Practicing postures with proper breathing helps the muscles relax by improving oxygen intake and circulation. Muscle relaxation directly relaxes the mind. When the mind begins to relax, muscles are able to further relax and stretch. This relieves built-up tension and stress. In order to relax the mind, we have to first take care of the body by practicing asanas. However, to fully relax the body, the mind has to develop a heightened awareness of the body. The **breath** is the dynamic link that unites the body and mind.

Yoga postures are the foundation for good health. Through the increase in circulation and liberation of prana, postures help control and regulate the endocrine (hormonal) system so that correct quantities of hormones are secreted by the various endocrine glands. Muscular, nervous, glandular, respiratory, excretory, and circulatory systems are also coordinated through postures along with their effects on the energy centers (chakras) and pressure points. The sympathetic and parasympathetic nervous systems are brought into a state of balance, helping the internal organs they control function properly.

Practicing postures also tones and beautifies the body by strengthening all the muscles, especially the spine where our nervous system resides. The strengthening of the spine and nervous system are essential to our ageless well-being. Regular practice of yoga asanas helps us regain youthfulness and feel and look younger.

The stretching of the muscles during the postures helps relax the body and alleviate the physical, mental, and emotional stress we encounter daily. Postures are effective in relieving back pains, headaches, insomnia, high and/ or low blood pressure, heart diseases, abdominal and lung ailments, and other stress-related ailments.

Ashok Jethanandani, publisher, India Currents magazine and a Bharatanatyam dancer, practices postures to ease his back pain. "When I started taking yoga classes with Vasanthi Bhat, I had a back injury that had not healed for four years. Sometimes my lower back would feel like it had a steel rod implanted along the spine. The back exercises that I had been doing until then had helped, but it was the hatha yoga routine that finally healed my back. The many postures and exercises Vasanthi Bhat taught me strengthened my back. The benefits of this yoga routine go beyond the physical. The breathing and meditation that go with the postures help me concentrate better, and I feel more energetic, relaxed, and upbeat on the days that I start with a few minutes of yoga."

Postures also calm and strengthen the mind. The key to attaining this peacefulness of mind is the integration of breathing with the asanas. Although we breathe naturally while holding the asanas, each asana has its own unique effect on the breath. Different asanas promote different types of breathing. Chest breathing becomes deeper in the backward bending and twisting positions when the chest is expanded. In the forward bending poses, breathing is centered in the thoracic cavity and the upper back. In the inverted poses, natural breathing becomes deeper and longer.

Rajiv Jaswa, a 9th grader, uses asanas to relieve headaches and improve concentration. "I first began attending Vasanthi's yoga classes after I was getting muscle tension headaches. I hoped yoga would terminate these pains. Yoga ended these, but that was just one minor benefit from yoga. The main benefit for me comes just before taking physical fitness tests in my physical education class, playing in football or basketball games, or engaging in any physical activity when I do pranayama - a yogic method of breathing. This enhances my ability to excel by improving my stamina and rejuvenating me. However, even these physical benefits do not match the psychological benefits yoga provides. I often do yoga before studying for major tests since it enhances my concentration. After doing even the simplest asanas, my stress no longer exists, and I am refreshed."

Postures are also one of the best preparations or foundations for good meditation. Holding the poses with steady, relaxed breathing in comfortable, non-exerting positions not only helps tone and strengthen the muscles, but also has a profound and immediate effect on our physical and mental well-being. The body feels totally relaxed and the mind calms down as the tension dissolves away. As the body, mind, and breath intertwine, a sense of unity and calmness surfaces, naturally leading to a peaceful meditative state. The true value of the asanas is realized when they are synchronized with proper breathing.

Often, I come across people who have been practicing yoga for many years and find the postures take a great deal of effort. They still have migraine headaches, back-pain, high blood pressure, heart diseases, abdominal ailments and other stress-related illnesses. Upon observing their technique, I noticed that the most important element - **CONSCIOUS BREATHING** - is missing in their practice. When we exert too much to attain an advanced level without giving attention to integrated breathing, the posture becomes useless, sometimes even harmful. When the breathing is irregular and not in tune with the pose, the body is not supplied with a sufficient amount of oxygen. This lack of oxygen further increases the tension in the already tense muscles and other parts of the body.

Amy Schlater from Seattle recalls, "After 10 years of practicing yoga with an aggressive, performance-oriented style with no breathing technique, my body was a mess. My nervous system was overly sensitive, and I had back pain and anxiety. I felt that the problem was the way I was practicing along with having no integrated breathing instruction. Under Vasanthi's video instruction, my energy and endurance returned, and yoga has been instrumental in my recovery from a heart rhythm disorder and back pain. Yoga is now my sustenance for daily living."

As shown, the lack of proper breathing leads to accumulated tension which causes stress. **Swami Satyananda Saraswati** addresses this topic in his teachings about tension. "Whether you think too much or you don't think at all, you accumulate tension. Whether you work physically or you do not work at all, you accumulate tension. Whether you sleep too much or not at all, you accumulate tension. And these tensions amass in the different layers of the human personality. They accumulate in the muscular, emotional, and mental systems. Therefore, tensions are of three types: muscular, mental, and emotional."

Tension is universal. It does not discriminate. People of all ages, from all walks of life experience some form of tension. In today's world, sometimes we can not prevent stressful situations; however, we can learn to manage and overcome them.

Tension is one cause of stress, but stress also surfaces as a reaction of the body and mind to difficult and challenging situations that have unpredictable and uncertain outcomes. This type of stress is caused when we are unable to gain control over the challenges; consequently, the body and the mind lose their balance. Feelings of helplessness and hopelessness ensue.

The following table lists some manifestations of the physical, mental, and emotional effects of stress that arise as a result of an imbalance and feelings of disparity. Depending on your genetic background and current health status, you may be susceptible to one or more of the following effects.

PHYSICAL EFFECTS	MENTAL/EMOTIONAL EFFECTS
Insomnia and fatigue	Anxiety and irritability
Nervous disorder	Lack of concentration
Headache	Anger
Cardiovascular disease	Depression
Gastrointestinal problems	Lack of interest in life
Lung ailments	Worthlessness
Obesity	Low self-esteem
Arthritis and/or rheumatism	

Table of Physical and Mental/Emotional Effects

How do stressful situations cause the symptoms mentioned above? Initially, when confronted with stressful situations there is an imbalance in the body's mechanism. The mind deviates towards the stressful situation and away from the body's natural balanced state. Breathing becomes rapid and short. Normal breathing becomes low priority and is overlooked. As a result, the biological systems become deficient in the oxygen needed to maintain general health, as well as balance emotional and mental states. This lack of oxygen throughout the body initially results in muscular tension. At this stage, the body, although still capable of coping, shows signs that it is being weakened and needs to be healed. If the tension is not relieved at this point, it accumulates and affects our well-being. Due to physical tension, we become irritable and anxious. Thus, the mind and emotions are affected again. The tension continues to accumulate until the body's systems are further impacted. As a result, physical and/or mental conditions manifest and cause emotional trauma.

This destructive cycle can be stopped in the beginning by practicing stretching and breathing techniques. Deep and relaxed breathing improves the quality of the blood circulating to all areas of the body. This supplies the muscles and organs with oxygen, preventing the accumulation of tension and the continuation of the vicious cycle! Remember, postures with controlled breathing are the backbone of our health and stress relief.

I still remember 21 years ago when I used to be under a great deal of stress; I suffered from migraine headaches and nervousness. My eyes were weak, and I was also overweight. I started yoga to relieve my migraine headaches and gain control of my weight. Soon the headaches disappeared, and I also lost weight. Not long after this, I even got rid of my glasses, which were used for nearsightedness. Later, as I got older, hemorrhoids appeared. Instead of blaming it on heredity, I increased the fiber intake in my diet and practiced the appropriate yoga techniques (rectal contractions and shoulder stand). Later, when I had problems with my thyroid gland, doctors suggested radiation treatment so that I would not have to constantly take medication. It was then that I remembered what the wise ancient yogis believed, "For every problem, there is a natural drug produced by our body." If the body can produce the ailments, the body is also capable of healing them. I continued doing yoga with this belief in mind and began integrating visualization and healing techniques (pranic healing) into my practice. That was it! It did not take very long to completely recover from my ailments. My hatha yoga practice (shoulder stand, plough, camel, cobra, spinal twist, alternate nostril breathing, and deep breathing) combined with conscious breathing and positive visualization helped me to alleviate my ailments.

When we are able to understand the connection between the body and mind, it does not take very long to learn to integrate yoga into our lives to overcome or prevent stress. With practice, we can learn to take complete control of our lives.

Dr. Theresa Frank, DDS, says, "I returned to the practice of yoga after a coincidence of events in my life left me with chronic pain in my shoulders and neck. I received whiplash from a car accident. I was caring for my 3-month old daughter, along with my 5-year old son. And I was returning to work part-time as a dentist. During that year of my life, I was unable to free myself of pain from the initial injury while continuing with my daily routine. I received medical care from a physician and from two different physical therapists. Neither the physical therapy nor the physician's treatment alleviated the pain. I began practicing yoga and found that after just a few exercises, the pain was gone. I attribute this to the relaxation and balance in the body and mind brought about by yogic breathing, stretching and strengthening exercises. For relief of my pain, yoga practice was more effective and more enjoyable than medications or physical therapy. I would recommend yoga for anyone, and I often do recommend it to my dental patients to relieve TMJ as well as head, shoulder, and neck pains. For this type of pain relief, I find that yoga is an easy, inexpensive, and effective treatment."

The reasons for practicing yoga are varied and differ from person to person. Some people just want to maintain their good health and stamina. Others have weak body parts they would like to strengthen or make more flexible. Still, others have ailments that they want to alleviate naturally. For whatever reason students come to my class, they experience the physical results and enjoy inner peace immediately. They say, "This is an hour of retreat. I feel I am in a different world." Many students mention that their spouses even encourage them to go to the class because they return so happy and cheerful for the entire day.

It is not necessary to practice yoga for many hours everyday. When pressed for time, you can even practice for as little as 5-15 minutes a day. Being able to enjoy and relax in the postures with deep concentration is far more important than how much time you spend doing the postures. Yoga can be practiced with even as few as one or two postures. These can be practiced at home, at work, or anywhere that is convenient. For example, some shoulder rotations and spinal twists can be adopted by people who have sedentary jobs. Similarly, people who are constantly on their feet can practice forward and backward bending poses to relieve mental fatigue.

Arvind Kumar, editor, India Currents magazine, says, "Over 10 years of working at a computer gave me carpal tunnel syndrome, a bad back, and weakening eyesight. Vasanthi Bhat showed me how with only 15 minutes a day, I could effectively reverse the symptoms and gain new levels of energy. Discovering Vasanthi Bhat and her unique style of yoga was a lifesaver."

It is also very reassuring to know that yoga postures can be practiced by anyone, at any age, under any physical condition, even by people who are bedridden. It is also important to know that people of all ages can practice for different reasons. For example, athletes and dancers can practice before and after their normal strenuous regime to stretch and strengthen their muscles, increase flexibility, and warm up or cool down. Housewives can use it to rejuvenate themselves and achieve mental peace. Executives and professionals can relieve their mental and physical fatigue. Children can practice to improve concentration in their activities. People confined to a bed can gently use it to recover their strength. Seniors can practice yoga to keep in shape, regain flexibility, and maintain strength and health.

Rose Mutzenburg started yoga when she was 64. She suffered from arthritis and could barely sit or get up. After six months of dedicated practice, she was able to gracefully assume difficult poses such as the shoulder stand and plough. Rose claimed that with yoga, her circulation, breathing, stamina, and memory improved tremendously. She is now able to keep busy with other physical activities such as water exercise, hiking, and travelling.

Yoga complements all types of activities including aerobics, walking, swimming, running, and many others. When practiced with certain poses like salutation to the sun, yoga can actually provide an invigorating cardio-vascular workout. It increases the energy level and helps stretch and tone the muscles. In addition, yoga can be used to warm up and cool down while preventing injuries and increasing flexibility.

Samantha Van Epps, an advanced yoga student, claims, "I have been taking yoga classes from Vasanthi for several years now, and I have come to appreciate the practice of hatha yoga in every way. I believe that warm-ups, postures, breathing, om chanting, and meditation take care of my needs in every way—physically, mentally, emotionally, and spiritually. Some warm-ups such as salutation to the sun, situps, and postures like locust, cobra, and bow are very powerful in exercising the heart and lungs. What more do I need except maybe to go for a nice walk as well? If I were to stop any activity in my life, yoga would be the last one."

So, it does not matter what other forms of exercise you do, how old you are, what state of health you are in, or what walk of life you come from. You just have to start where you are, practice the poses and breathing that are appropriate to your situation, relax, and enjoy yourself.

It is extremely important to know the benefits of the asanas. For example, the pose of the moon stretches and tones the spine, stimulates the digestive system, increases circulation towards the head, and relaxes the leg muscles. This provides relief from back aches, abdominal ailments, sinus congestion, headaches, and arthritis in the legs. Healing can be accelerated if you direct and focus your mind to an affected area. While doing the postures, visualize the energy or prana being directed to affected areas and enhance it's healing powers with positive, kind, and loving thoughts.

Carolyn Garbarino, technical editor, says, "I have Chronic Fatigue Immune Dysfunction Syndrome and do not have the stamina for aerobic exercise. I sought yoga class as a way to get non-aerobic exercise to release stress and perhaps heal. After studying with Vasanthi for more than a year, I have improved my stamina. When I first started yoga, I could not do one hour of asanas. Now I can do an hour of asanas with energy to spare. I have lost seven pounds and have better muscle tone than at any time in six years of having this disease. I stay with Vasanthi's class because I feel a great sense of well-being afterward. Her meditation lectures always yield some important bit of information that I need to improve my life right now."

For specific ailments, the regular practice of even one posture can provide tremendous benefits.

Nikhil Deshmukh, a 10-year old, practices yoga to relieve asthma. "One day during physical education, my classmates and I had to run the mile. After the run, I was wheezing and about to go to the school nurse for my inhaler. Instead, I thought (as Vasanthi teaches) of using yoga to help my breathing. I did the matsya asana (fish pose) which stopped the wheezing and prevented an asthma attack."

Do not ever get discouraged by thinking that your body is not flexible enough. Often people say that they are not able to bend and touch their toes or sit in the lotus position. They wonder how they can practice yoga. Yoga is not practiced to stretch your body with force by twisting and performing advanced poses. Rather, it is an art in which you listen to your body and practice accordingly without comparing yourself to anyone or any standards.

Prochy Sethna, an engineer, started slowly and practiced patiently. She diligently took time to stretch and did not compare herself to anyone. She attended classes rain or shine and noticed steady improvement. Although it took her two years to develop mastery, she has been experiencing the marvelous results for the past ten years.

Below is a summary of the types of postures and their benefits. It is advisable to always begin your yoga practice with a few warm-up exercises to prevent muscle pull and stiffness.

TYPE OF POSTURES	BENEFITS OF POSTURES
Warm-up exercises	Relax the tense and stiff muscles, making them less susceptible to muscle pull. Help relieve constipation and intestinal gases. Aid in the release of acids in the joints, which can cause arthritic stiffness and rheumatic pain.
Standing poses[1]	Improve concentration, balance, and poise. Provide a stretch for the whole body.
Forward bending poses	Stretch and tone the spinal nerves, making the back muscles strong and supple. Compress and massage the abdominal organs. Increase circulation towards the face and head, thereby improving eyesight, memory, and concentration.
Backward bending poses	Relieve back pain. Prevent slipped discs. Stretch the abdominal muscles. Strengthen the heart and lungs. Help prevent and alleviate heart and lung ailments as well as breast cancer. Tone the arm, neck, and facial muscles, providing the effect of a massage. Stimulate thyroid glands.
Inverted poses	Increase blood flow to the head; nourish brain cells. Improve thinking power, concentration, and stamina. Relieve stress, headache, and sinus congestion. Help normalize thyroid functioning. Relieve lung ailments. Regain youthfulness. Improve facial texture and eyesight. Prevent hair loss. Help control and evenly distribute body weight.
Spinal twist poses	Exercise the spine and trunk. Loosen the spinal column and stimulate the related nerves. Massage abdominal organs and chest areas. Relax the heart and lungs. Also aid in preventing breast cancer. Massage upper back, shoulders, arms, and neck. Relieve arthritis and rheumatic pain.

[1] Standing poses can be practiced separately when you are pressed for time.

THINGS TO KNOW BEFORE PRACTICING YOGA ASANAS

- Practice yoga with utmost concentration. Even a few moments of focused, mindful practice can be very beneficial.

- Practice yoga in a clean, well-ventilated area. Although the hours during sunrise and sunset are ideal, you may choose a comfortable time that suites your schedule. Also, if possible, try to practice after a shower or bath when your skin pores are clean and open. This intensifies the effects of yoga and allows you to absorb prana better, thereby improving stamina and strengthening the immune system. However, there is no harm in not taking a shower or practicing at other times of the day.

- Wear loose, comfortable clothing.

- Practice yoga on an empty stomach. When the stomach is full, the mind loses its concentration. Also, practicing yoga draws blood away from the digestive process and may cause indigestion and cramps.

- Remember to empty your bladder and/or bowels prior to yoga practice, so it is easy to practice the asanas that compress the stomach and abdomen. Warm-ups and deep breathing can be practiced to relieve constipation. Drinking warm or hot water also helps.

- On menstrual days, women should avoid practicing postures that compress the abdominal region, such as preliminary leg pull, shoulder stand, and plough. Less compressing poses, such as the camel, pose of the moon, standing poses, and pranayama techniques can be practiced to help relieve exhaustion and cramps.

- Before beginning your yoga practice, perform a few warm-up exercises to prepare your body and prevent unnecessary muscle pulls.

- Never use force or strain while practicing yoga. Close your eyes and listen to your body while holding the poses. It is natural to feel stiff at first. With regular practice, you will notice significant progress.

- Check the end of this chapter for a list of suggested routines.

WARM-UPS

Warm-ups are movements that help loosen the muscles and joints in order to prevent muscle pulls and prepare the body for the asanas. They are also known as Pawan Muktasana ('pawan' means wind and 'mukta' means release).

They are called wind release exercises because they stretch, compress, and massage various areas of the body to release and prevent toxic buildups which manifest as stomach acidity, heartburn, indigestion, flatulence, joint pains, arthritis, rheumatism, and other disturbances. Often, the built-up toxins are released as gas, while the other toxins dissipate throughout the body.

These warm-ups are highly recommended for people who have not practiced any form of stretching. Depending on your needs and physical condition, practice some or all of the warm-ups before practicing any asanas. Also, increase or decrease the duration of your warm-ups as you desire. For example, to condition the hips and other areas below the waist, spend extra time practicing the cycling routine. To condition the neck muscles, allow more time for the leg lock warm-up routine. If you have sore or injured muscles, reduce your warm-up time or eliminate the routines that aggravate the injured area. During all the warm-up movements, breathe normally unless otherwise mentioned.

ANKLE ROTATION AND FLEX

Practice

Sit with your legs slightly apart and extended in front of you. Let your arms rest at your side. Rotate your feet inward and then outward several times, while your legs remain stationary. You can also practice rotating each foot separately. After rotating your feet several times in both directions, flex your feet forward and then backward 5-10 times.

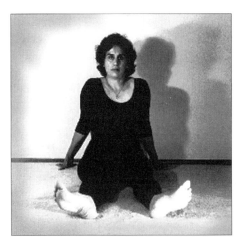 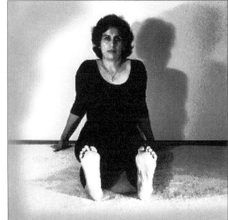

Benefits

Strengthens the ankles, calves, and feet. Provides relief for arthritic stiffness and rheumatic pain. Serves as a preparatory exercise for people who cannot sit on their heels in a kneeling position or for those practicing aerobic exercises.

HAND AND WRIST STRETCH

Practice

Sitting or standing, extend your arms straight in front of you at shoulder level. Make a tight fist with your hands closing your fingers over your thumbs. Rotate your wrists inward and outward, 5-10 times.

Release your hands and stretch your fingers as far out as possible. Repeat 5-10 times.

With your hands open and palms facing down, move your palms up and down about the wrist joints. Repeat 5-10 times.

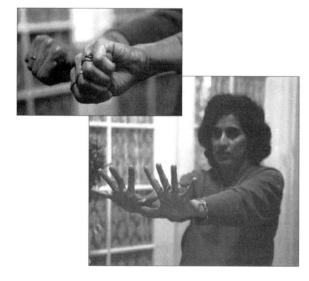
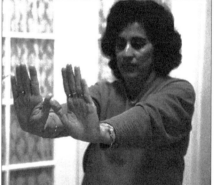

Benefits

Strengthens the wrist joints, arms, and fingers. Provides relief for arthritic stiffness, rheumatic pain, tendinitis, and carpal tunnel syndrome. Beneficial for typists, body sculptors, and weight lifters.

SPLITS

Practice

Sit straight with your legs apart, palms resting on your legs. Breathing out, bend forward. Relax in this position while breathing naturally for 5-10 seconds. Relax your neck muscles and lower your head gently as you stretch further. Hold this position while breathing normally for 15-30 seconds.

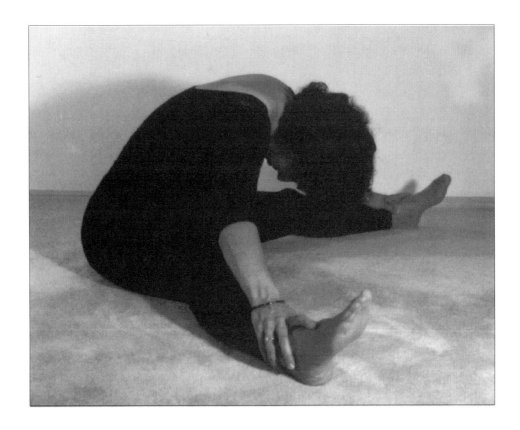

You may rest your arms out in front of you, bending slightly at the elbows. Stretch further if your body permits. Maintain normal breathing.

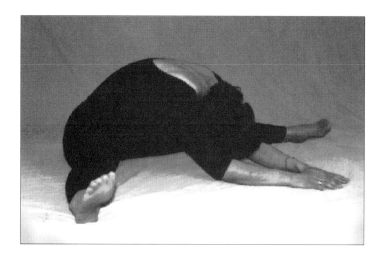

Proceed to this variation with caution. Using force is extremely dangerous for the spine and hamstrings. Hold your toes while resting your head.

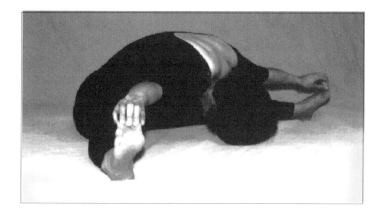

Benefits

Loosens the neck, upper back, spine, hips, hamstrings, and groin.

CHURNING THE MILL (Chakki Chalana)

Practice

Sit with your legs extended in front of you. Straighten your arms in front of you at shoulder level and interlock your thumbs. Breathing out and breathing in, move your body forward and backward respectively. Make 5-10 circular movements clockwise, and then counterclockwise.

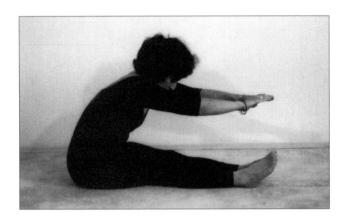

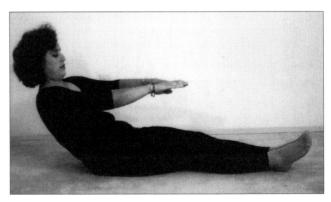

Benefits

Soothes and stretches the spine and hips. Tones the arms, upper back, shoulder muscles, and hamstrings. Improves digestion. Relieves constipation, cramps, and stomach acid pains.

HIP STRETCH

Practice

Sit straight with your legs apart. Hold the side of your right leg with your left arm. Turn your body from the waist up, raise your right arm, and stretch as much as you can. Fix your gaze on your raised palm as you breathe naturally for 10-15 seconds. You may try to hold your toes by twisting your upper body as shown in the inset. Switch sides and repeat this sequence as shown on the next page.

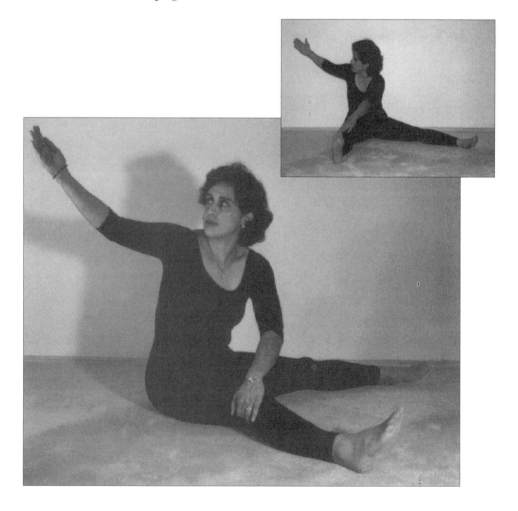

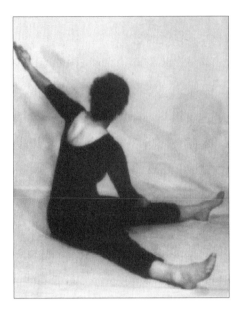

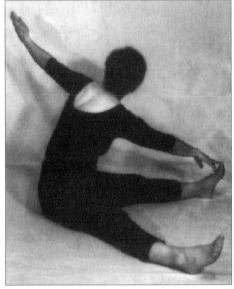

Benefits

Relaxes the neck, upper back, shoulders, and arms. Tones hip muscles, hamstrings, lower back, and trims the waistline. Strengthens the heart and lungs. Relieves arthritic stiffness and provides a good warm-up for a stiff body.

BUTTERFLY STRETCHES

Practice A (Half Butterfly)

Sit with your legs extended in front of you. Bend your left leg at the knee, and rest your foot on top of your right thigh as close to your groin as possible. Holding your foot and knee, move your left leg up and down, as a butterfly flutters its wings, for 30 seconds.

Then, keeping your leg bent, try to push your left knee towards the floor as much as possible. Repeat the same movement using your right leg.

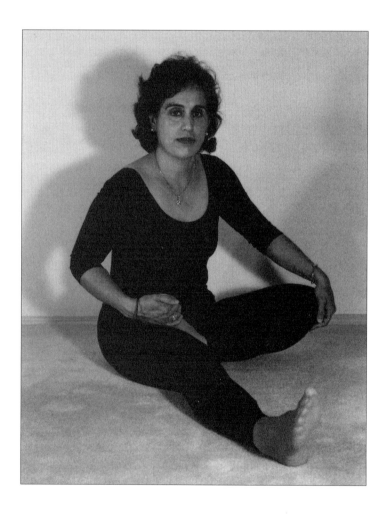

Practice B (Full Butterfly)

Sit with both legs bent at the knees, while bringing the soles of your feet together. Interlock your fingers around your feet and pull your feet close to your body. Move your knees up and down as a butterfly flutters its wings, for 30 seconds. Then, try to push your knees towards the floor and hold for a few moments.

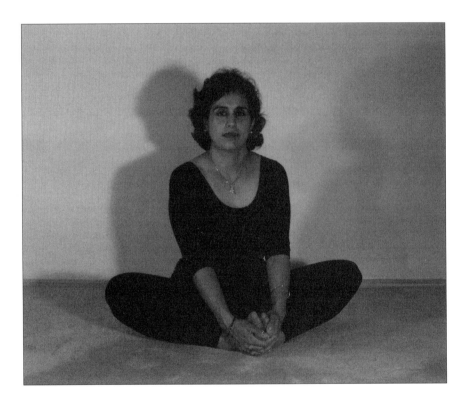

Benefits

Strengthens and loosens the hip joints, groin, and leg muscles. Also prepares the body for sitting in the lotus (padmasana) position.

CYCLING

Practice

Lie flat on your back with your hands by your side, palms facing down. Lift both legs and slowly move your legs in a forward cycling motion for 15-30 rounds, while breathing naturally. Rest for a few seconds, before proceeding with backward cycling movements.

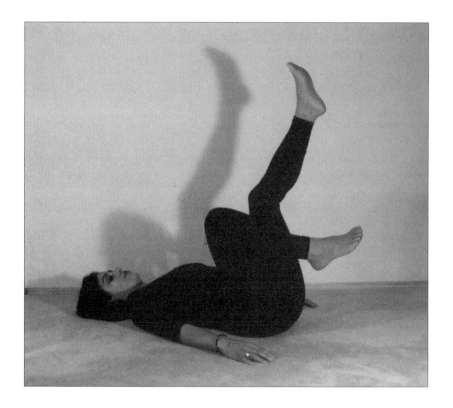

Benefits

Strengthens and conditions the lower part of the abdomen, lower back, hips, groin, thighs, and knees. Provides relief for lower back pain.

LEG LOCK

Practice

Lie flat on your back. Bend your left leg at the knee and bring it towards your chest. Interlock your fingers around your bent leg, between your calf and knee. As you breathe out (pulling in your stomach), lift your head and upper back. (As the practice becomes easier, try to hold this position while breathing naturally.) You may also allow your forehead to touch your knee. Breathing in, rest your head on the floor. This is one round. Repeat 3-5 times. Continue this sequence with your right leg. Afterwards you may advance to the two-leg lock, as shown.

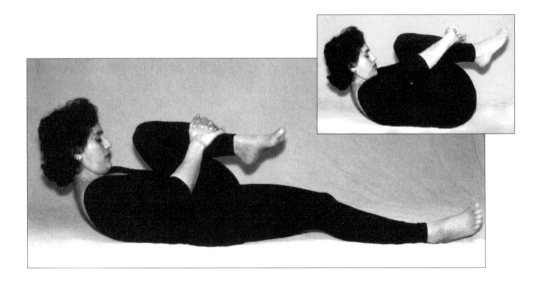

Benefits

Massages and tones the neck, upper back, shoulders, and spine, and releases upper-body tension. Tones and massages the facial muscles. Provides mental relaxation. Helps prevent and treat whiplash. Improves digestion. Relieves constipation, cramps, and other abdominal ailments. Provides a gentle stretch to the sciatic nerves and hips.

LYING TWIST

Practice

Lie flat on your back, with both legs bent at the knees, soles resting on the floor, arms at your sides. Cross your right leg over your left and roll over to the left as shown in the inset. Stretch your arms upwards and turn your face toward the opposite side. Hold this position for a comfortable length of time while breathing naturally with your eyes closed. Repeat this pose on the opposite side, with your left leg crossed over your right.

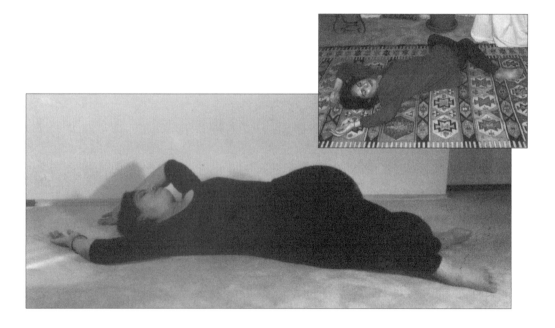

Benefits

Provides a great stretch for the hips, sciatic nerves, lower back, chest, neck, and arms. Encourages deep breathing, providing extra relaxation and exercise for the heart and lungs. Helps prevent breast cancer by increasing circulation, while stretching the chest area. Relieves physical, mental, and emotional tension.

SIT UPS to BOAT STRETCH

If you have stiffness or pain in your neck or back, practice this posture carefully.

Practice

Lie flat with your legs bent at the knee, arms resting at your side. As you breathe out, lift your head, upper back, and arms, and reach out towards your knees as far as possible. Breathing in, rest your upper body and head on the floor. Repeat 5-10 times.

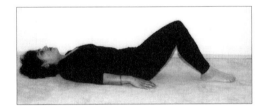

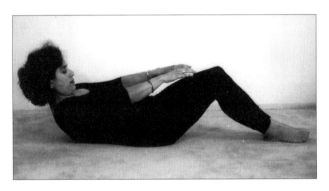

With practice, you will gradually be able to lift your upper body with ease.

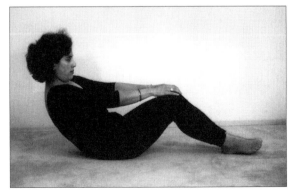

As the practice becomes easier, straighten your legs after lifting your upper body. Breathe naturally and hold the position comfortably. As your practice advances you will be able to raise your legs further in a vertical position and hold the position for 10-15 seconds.

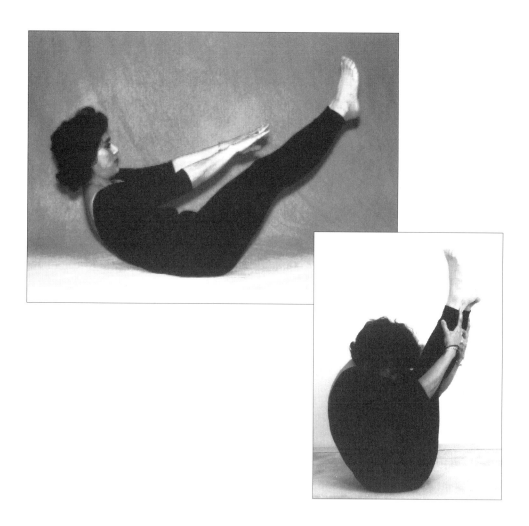

Benefits

Provides a great stretch for the spine, back, hips, and neck, while strengthening and firming the abdominal muscles.

NECK MOVEMENTS

Practice

Stand or sit with your back straight. Slowly look up as you breathe in. Then, slowly look down as you breathe out. Rotate your head several times clockwise and then counterclockwise. Repeat as often as needed.

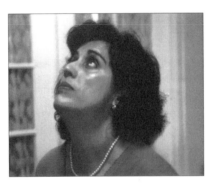
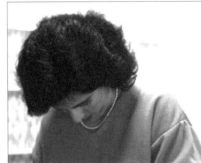
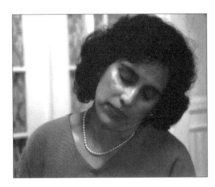
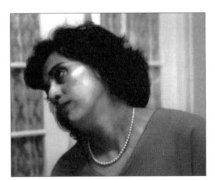

Benefits

Provides immediate relief for a stiff and tensed neck and upper back. Also, relieves mental fatigue by stretching and soothing the muscles connected to the brain.

SHOULDER SOCKET ROTATION

Practice

Sit or stand straight with your feet slightly apart. Rest your fingers on your shoulders, elbows pointing forward. Then, rotate your arms and shoulders, making circular motions at the elbows, several times. Repeat these movements in the opposite direction.

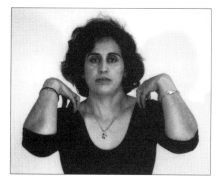
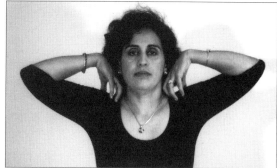

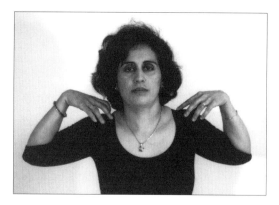

Benefits

Releases tension from the upper back, shoulder joints, and neck, and tones the corresponding muscles. Beneficial for weight lifters and athletes.

TRIANGLE STRETCH (Trikonasana)

Practice

Stand with feet about two feet apart, arms extended to the side at the shoulder level as shown.

Breathing out, bend towards the left. Breathing in, move back to the upright position. Breathing out, bend towards the right. Breathing in, return to the upright position. You can either repeat 3-4 times or hold the stretch on both sides, while breathing normally.

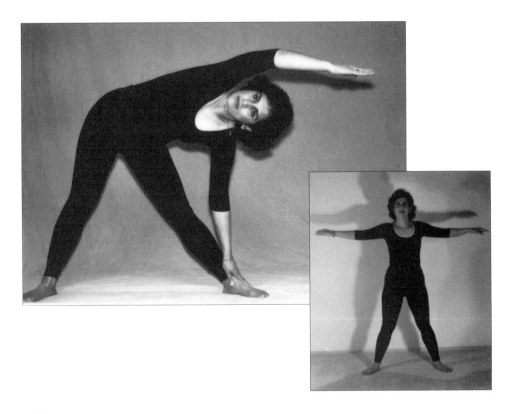

Benefits

Tones the muscles of the neck, shoulders, back, arms, legs, and hips. Provides excellent relief for back pain and nervous tension.

TOE AND BACK STRETCH (Padasana)

Practice

Stand on your toes. Raise both arms. Interlocking your fingers, stretch up as much as possible. Breathe deeply for about 10 seconds. While breathing out, bend forward at the waist until the trunk and arms are parallel to the floor. Hold this position for 15-30 seconds. Breathing in, come back to the standing position. Repeat as needed.

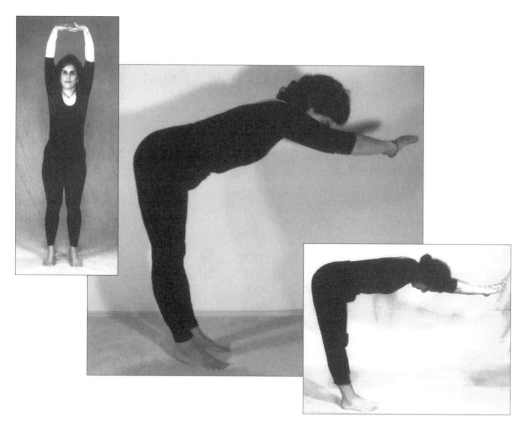

Benefits

Provides immediate relief for physical and mental tension. Stretches the entire body from the toes to the fingers, including the spine, arms, neck, hamstrings, and feet.

WARRIOR POSE (Veerabhadrasana)

Practice

Begin by standing with your feet apart. Gently turn your right foot so it is perpendicular to the left. Raise your arms and arch backward while bending your left leg. Breathe slowly and deeply for a comfortable length of time. Repeat the sequence by turning to the opposite side.

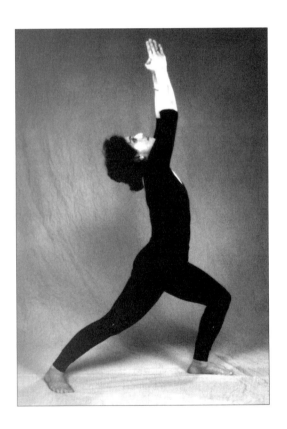

Benefits

Tones the arms, neck, shoulders, biceps, hips, quadriceps, legs, and calves. Relieves tension from the chest muscles and releases energy from the base of the spine. Soothes the mind by uplifting the emotions.

FEET AND PALM STRETCH (Pada Hastasana)

Practice

Stand with the feet slightly apart. Stretch both the arms straight up. Breathing out, bend forward until your palms or fingers touch the floor or as much as you can comfortably stretch. Breathe naturally as you hold the position for 15-30 seconds. Breathing in, come out of the position. If you are unable to touch the floor, grasp your wrist behind your legs as shown. You may bend your legs slightly at the knee.

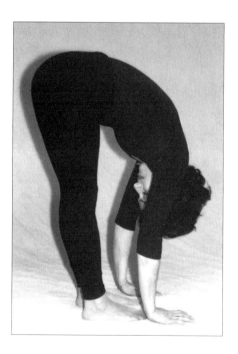 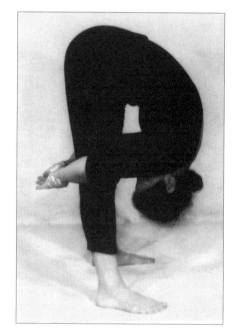

Benefits

Provides a good stretch from the feet to the palms. Improves general circulation. Eases mental fatigue. Relaxes the eyes and brings a glow to the face.

ARM AND LEG STRETCH (Nataraja Asana)

Practice

Stand straight. Bend your right leg at the knee and hold your ankle. Lift your left arm above your shoulder. Gently lift your knee while arching your back and looking up. It is perfectly allright to use support for balance. Breathing naturally, hold the position for 5-10 seconds. You can also bend forward as shown. Repeat the identical movements with the opposite leg and arm.

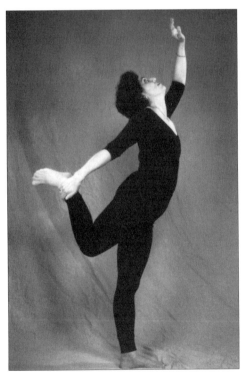
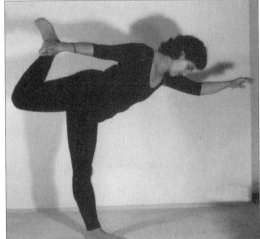

Benefits

Provides a good stretch for the neck, face, eyes, arms, chest, abdominal area, hips, legs, and spine.

ONE LEG STRETCH (Eka Padasana)

Practice

Stand straight. Balancing on one leg, lift and stretch your other leg backward while extending your arms in front of you to form a T-shaped pose. Breathing naturally, hold the position for 10-30 seconds. Repeat the same movements, balancing on the opposite leg.

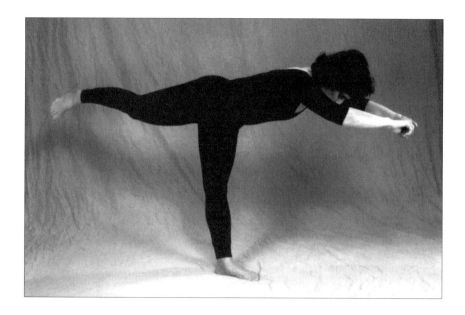

Benefits

Conditions the legs and hips, providing the effects of weight lifting. Tones the hamstrings, spine, and arms. An easy technique for spinal alignment.

HALF LOTUS TREE POSE (Ardha Padmasana Vrikshasana)

Practice

Stand straight. Bend your left leg so your foot rests on the opposite thigh.
Lift your arms up bringing your palms together. Hold the position for 10-
30 seconds.

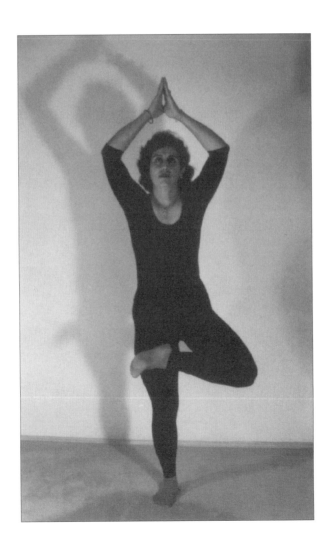

Bend forward as you breathe out. Breathe naturally in this position for 10-30 seconds. Breathing in, come out of the position. Repeat the same procedure with the right leg.

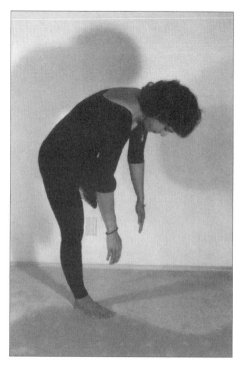 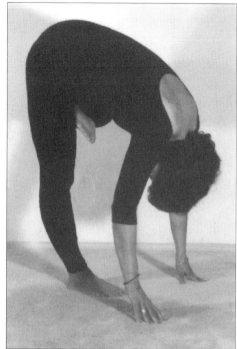

Benefits

Tones the hips and quadriceps. Provides flexibility to the hamstrings and spine. Improves overall circulation.

DOUBLE ANGLE STRETCH (Dwikonasana)

Practice

Stand straight with your feet a few inches or about one foot apart. Clasp your hands behind your back, while straightening your arms. Move your arms slightly away from your body. Breathe in as you bend backward. Pause for a moment. Breathe out as you bend forward, keeping your arms straight. Breathe naturally while holding this position. You may stretch your arms further as shown on the next page. Breathing in, come up, release your hands, and relax.

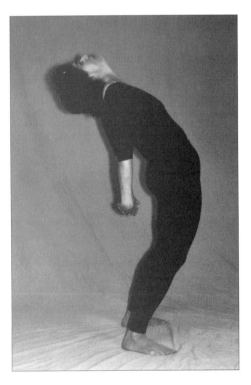 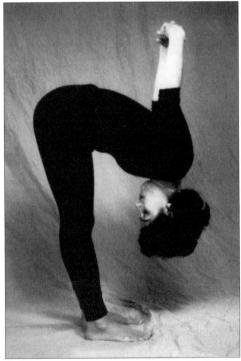

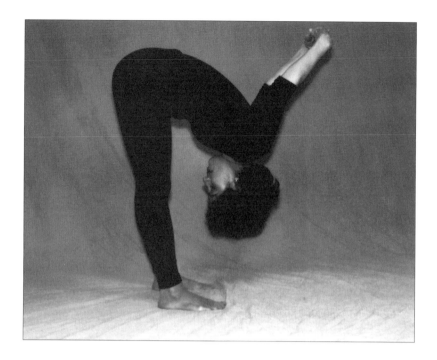

Benefits

Stretches and tones the spine, arms, shoulders, upper back, neck, and hamstrings. Relaxes the eyes and brings a glow to the face. Quickly relieves mental fatigue by improving blood circulation towards the face and head. Extremely beneficial for quick revitalization.

ABDOMINAL LIFT (Udiyana Bandha)

Practice

Stand with your legs shoulder width apart. Bend slightly and rest your palms on your knees. Breathe in. As you breathe out, pull your stomach in as much as possible.

While holding the breath (do not breathe in), gently pull your stomach in further as shown on the next page. Notice, you will have to tighten the chest and arms while you are trying to pull your stomach in. Hold the position for a few seconds. Breathing in comes naturally deeper as you release your stomach muscles. Repeat 2-3 times.

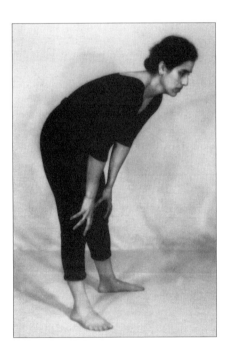

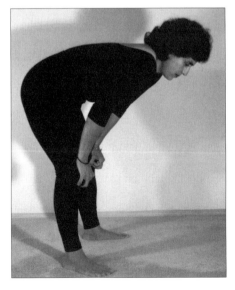

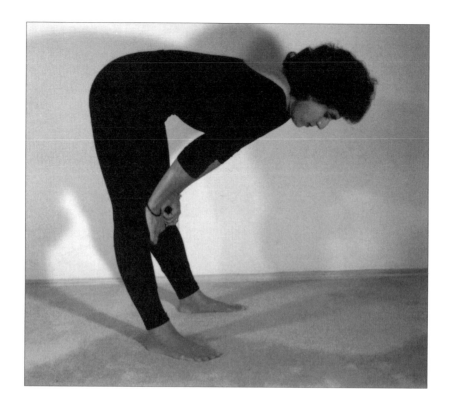

Benefits

Stimulates intestinal activity and strengthens the abdominal area. Helps prevent colon cancer, fibroids, and other abdominal ailments. Reduces excess fat from the abdominal area. Improves digestion and relieves constipation.

SALUTATION TO THE SUN (Surya Namaskara)

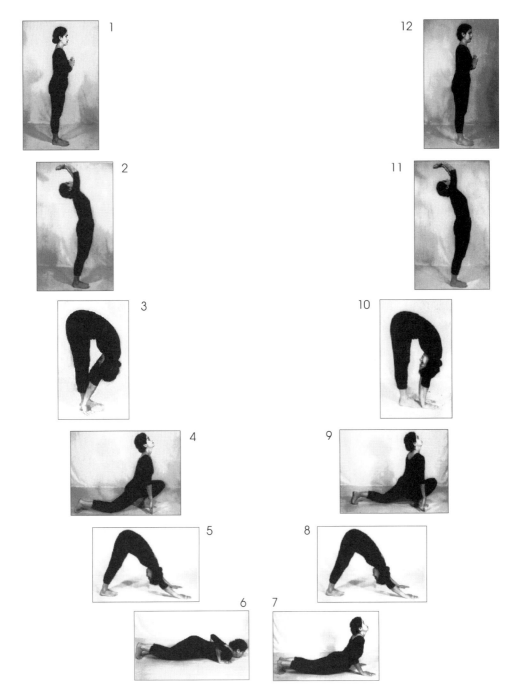

Practice

The salutation to the sun[2] consists of two sets of the 12-step movements shown on the previous page. In the first set of 12 movements, move your right leg back and forth in steps 4 and 9. In the second set of 12 movements, move your left leg back and forth in steps 4 and 9. One round of salutation to the sun refers to two complete sets of the 12-step movements.

Step 1.
Salute (Namaskara)

Breathe out as you begin the pose.

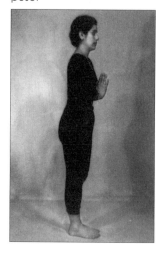

Step 2.
Raised arm pose
(Hasta uttanasana)

Breathing in, raise your arms and bend backward.

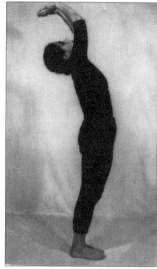

Step 3.
Palm and feet stretch
(Pada hastasana)

Breathing out, pull your stomach in and bend forward. You may bend your legs at the knee if necessary.

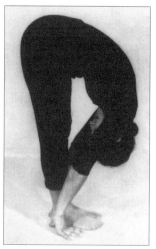

[2]Ancient people had great respect for the sun. In its original form, Indian yogis used to practice salutation to the sun in a quiet place, preferably outside, at sunrise, facing the east after their morning bath to revitalize, energize, and increase stamina. Although you may not be able to practice outdoors in front of the rising sun, you may practice in front of an open door, window, or any suitable location.

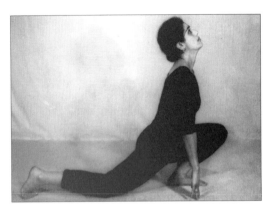

Step 4.

Equestrian pose
(Ashwa sanchalanasana)

Breathing in, move your right leg backward. You may rest your arms on your knees or raise your arms above your head as in the warrior pose.

Step 5.

Mountain pose (Parvatasana)

Breathing out, move your left leg back and raise your hips. Try not to bend your legs at the knees to rest your heels fully. Instead, you may allow your heels to be slightly raised.

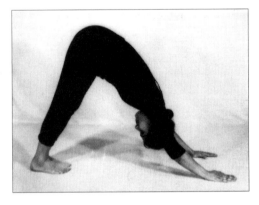

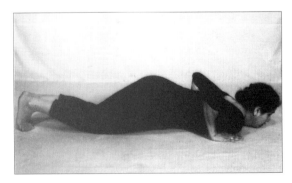

Step 6.

Eight-limb salute
(Ashtanga namaskara)

Breathing naturally or holding your breath, lower your body resting your knees, chest, and chin on the floor.

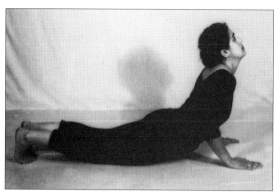

Step 7.
Cobra (Bhujangasana)
Breathing in, raise your upper body.

Step 8.
Mountain pose (Parvatasana)
Breathing out, assume the mountain pose.

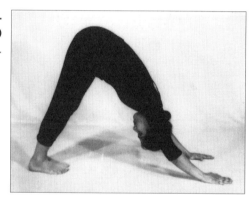

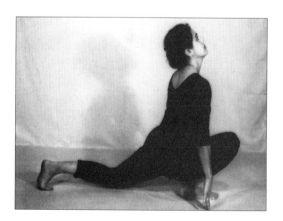

Step 9.
Equestrian pose
(Ashwa sanchalanasana)
Breathing in, move your right leg forward.

Step 10.
Palm and feet stretch (Pada hastasana)
Breathing out, pull your stomach in, and bend forward. You may rest your palms in front of your feet.

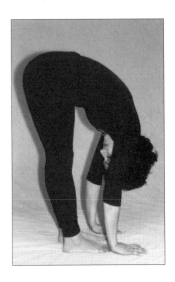

Step 11.
Raised arm pose (Hasta uttanasana)
Breathing in, raise your arms and bend backwards.

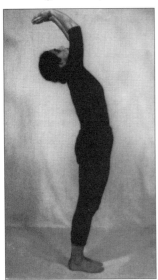

Step 12.
Salute (Namaskara)
Breathe out as you lower your arms.

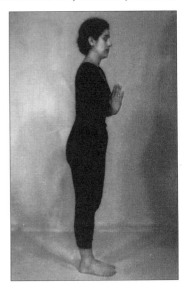

Repeat the 12 steps to complete one round, moving the left leg in steps 4 and 9. Practice 2-5 rounds. In an advanced stage, you may hold the position in some or all the steps to experience an intense stretch. Breathe naturally while holding the positions.

Benefits

Salutation to the sun is a dynamic workout which not only stretches and tones the whole body, but energizes the entire system with the synchronized breathing. It only takes 3-5 minutes of practice to make you feel strong, energetic, and wonderful.

Improves concentration and stamina, and encourages deep breathing. Stretches and strengthens the feet, hamstrings, spine, hips, neck, and arms. The intense breathing and chest expansion strengthen the lungs and help alleviate the effects of allergy, asthma, and the common cold. Provides a good cardiovascular workout and a feeling of well-being. Prevents hair loss by nourishing the scalp. Improves circulation to the face, adding extra glow. Tones and beautifies the body. Helps in the proper distribution of body weight.

CORPSE RELAXATION (Shavasana)

Practice

Lie flat on your back, with your arms at your side and legs apart. Adjust your position to be comfortable. Bring your awareness towards your breath. Feel your breath flow in and out through your nostrils for about 15 seconds. Then start breathing deeply. Make sure to compress your stomach while prolonging your exhalations. Relax your stomach muscles and breathe in upward while expanding your chest. Continue to breathe deeply for about 2 minutes to relieve tension. Then focus on your natural breath and relax your entire body from head to toe. Refer to Chapter 2 on pranayama for detailed instructions on corpse relaxation.

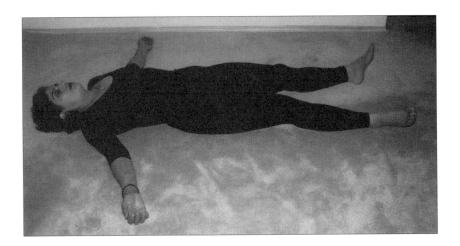

Benefits

Relaxes the entire body (all the muscles which are exercised during the warm-ups). Releases physical, mental, and emotional tension. Helps the practitioner perform asanas with ease.

ASANAS

Asanas are postures in which you remain steady and comfortable with relaxed breathing. When practicing the asanas, remember to close your eyes and listen to your body. Depending on the time available, stay in the asana anywhere from a few seconds to as long as you feel comfortable. For quick relaxation, hold the position for 15-30 seconds. For conditioning the muscles and for therapeutic purposes, stay in the asana for about 60 seconds. You should immediately come out of a pose the moment you experience uneasiness. Often, feelings of uneasiness arise naturally as a response to the stress and anxiety stored in your body. These feelings can come up for anyone at any time during the postures, even for people who have been practicing yoga for many years. However, with practice, the feelings of uneasiness occur less frequently and with diminished effect.

Breathing properly while performing the asanas is also very important. During forward bending poses, be sure to breathe out as you pull the stomach in. Breathe in as you come out of the pose. During most backward bending poses, breathe in as you assume the pose. Breathe out as you come out of the pose. Breathe freely or naturally while holding all the positions to ensure good circulation and revitalization.

For beginners, it is best to repeat each asana 2-3 times, resting in between as needed. After some practice, you will begin to feel comfortable and relaxed in the asana. When you reach this point, there is no need to repeat the postures. Instead, try to hold each asana for a longer period. Keep in mind, there is no harm in repeating your favorite postures as often as you like. Some postures have several variations which are listed in the order of most basic to advanced.

When you become comfortable practicing the asanas at an advanced level, you can practice deep breathing and meditation while holding certain asanas, such as pose of the moon, shoulder stand, plough, turtle, and bowing pose. Deep breathing and meditation intensifies the benefits for the internal parts and releases any built-up tension. Chapter 3 on meditation provides more information on healing by visualization (pranic healing).

POSE OF THE MOON (Shashankasana)

An easy meditative pose and a great emotional, mental, and muscular stress reliever!

Practice

Note: If you have an injured knee, practice this and the turtle pose with caution.

Sit on your heels with feet flat as shown. Breathing in deeply, lift your arms straight above your head. Breathing out, pull your stomach in, lower your trunk, and rest your forehead on the floor. Close your eyes and breathe naturally for 30-60 seconds. Breathing in, slowly come back to the sitting position.

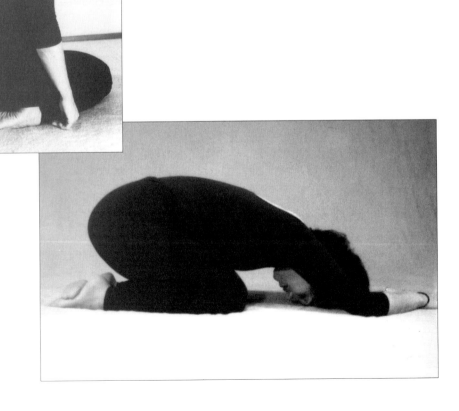

If you find it difficult to sit on your heels, you may raise your hips while sliding your arms forward and depressing your spine. This variation also relieves back pain and increases spinal flexibility.

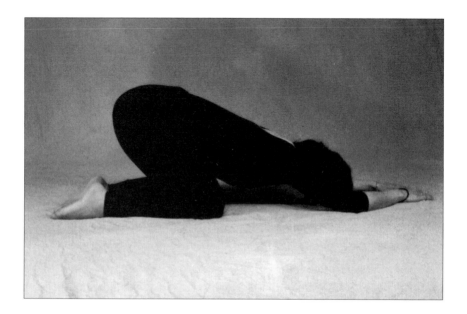

Benefits

Stretches and tones the spine, hips, and sciatic nerves. Relieves back pain. Relaxes the heart muscles. Compresses the stomach and abdominal area; activates digestion; strengthens the abdominal and pelvic areas; helps alleviate and prevent acidity, cramps of any kind, and intestinal or toxic growths. Increases circulation to the head and face, alleviating mental fatigue and tension headaches. In addition, improves eye sight and facial texture.

TURTLE POSE (Kurmasana)

A very soothing pose for the mind and soul.

Practice

Sit on your heels. While breathing out, pull your stomach in and rest either your head or forehead on the floor. Rest your arms at your side or hold your wrists at the back as shown on the next page. Breathe naturally. Remain in the position for 30-60 seconds. Breathing in, come out of the pose.

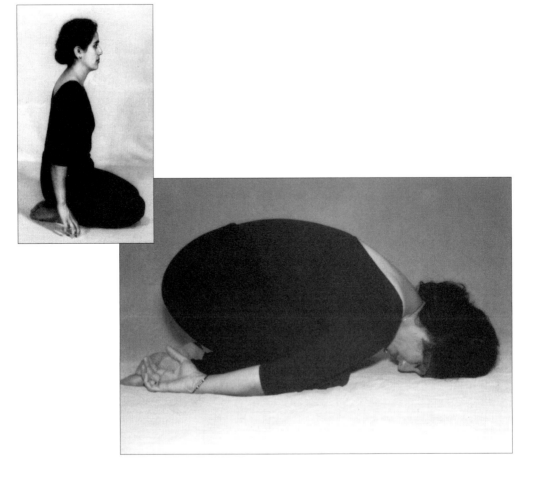

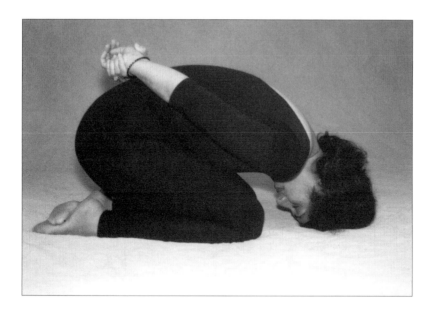

Benefits

Increases flexibility of the entire spine, hips, and neck muscles. Tones the spine, hips, and sciatic nerves. Provides great relief for back pains. Relaxes the heart muscles. Emphasizes thoracic breathing; exercises the lungs. The compression on the stomach and abdominal areas activates digestion; strengthens the abdominal and pelvic areas; helps alleviate and prevent acidity, cramps of any kind, and intestinal or toxic growths. Increases blood supply to the head and face, relieving tension headaches and mental fatigue. Enhances memory and concentration. Improves eye sight and brings a glow to the face.

BOWING POSE (Pranamasana)

An easy meditative pose and a great sinus congestion reliever!

Practice

Sit on your heels.

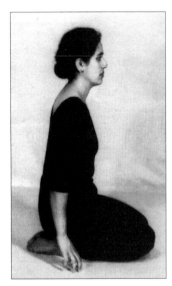

While breathing out, lift your hips and rest the top of your head on the floor. Rest your arms at your side. Breathe naturally while holding the position for 30-60 seconds. Breathing in, come up and relax.

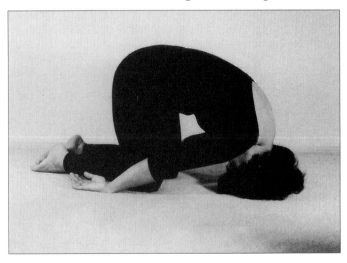

Variation

Adopt this variation for strengthening shoulders, arms, wrist joints, and chest muscles.

Note: You may perform pose of the moon, turtle, and bowing poses in a continuous sequence.

Interlock your fingers. Breathe in as you stretch backwards.

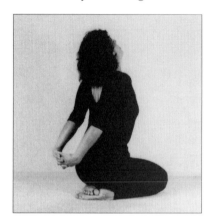

Breathe out as you bend forward. Breathe naturally in this position for 30-60 seconds. Breathing in, come out of the pose.

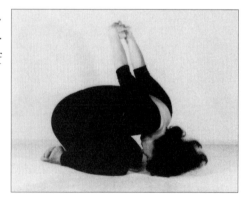

Benefits

Increases blood circulation towards the head and provides immediate mental relaxation. Improves memory, eye sight, and complexion. Prevents hair loss. Effectively relieves sinus congestion. Improves concentration, memory, and will power.

MOUNTAIN POSE (Parvatasana)

A quick body stretch and energizer!

Practice

Sit on your heels with your toes bent. Bend forward resting your palms on the floor. Raise your torso while straightening your legs and arms. Breathe normally. If you have carpal tunnel syndrome, make a fist to ease your discomfort. Try to rest your heels on the floor as shown in the inset. Do not use force or strain to rest your heels. Using force may cause harm to your hamstring muscles. Breathe normally in the pose for 15-30 seconds. Bend your legs at the knees and return to the sitting position.

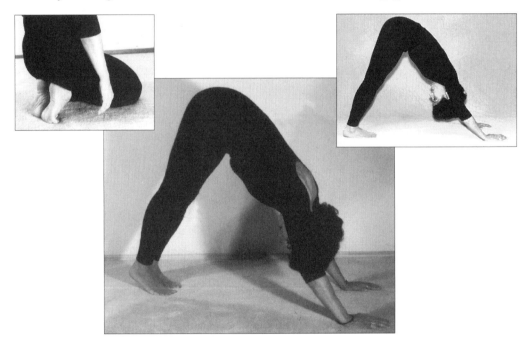

Benefits

Provides a great, energizing stretch for the whole body, including feet, ankles, hamstrings, spine, arms, and wrist joints. Provides immense relief from carpal tunnel syndrome, arthritis, and tendinitis. Increases blood circulation to the brain, relieving mental fatigue.

PRELIMINARY HEADSTAND

A great relief for physical and mental fatigue.

Practice

Sit on your heels with toes bent, as in the mountain pose. Kneel down, as in the bowing pose. Interlock your fingers behind your head and slowly straighten your legs. Breathe normally. Hold this pose for 15-30 seconds. Be sure to balance your weight evenly between your arms, head, and legs.

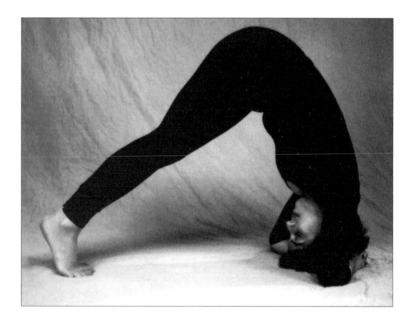

Benefits

Increases blood circulation to the head, relieving mental fatigue. Improves memory and concentration. Relaxes the eyes and brings a glow to the face. Provides a great, energizing stretch for the whole body, including feet, ankles, hamstrings, spine, arms, and wrist joints.

CAT (Marjariasana)

An easy pose for back pain relief.

Practice

Get down on your knees. Rest your palms below your shoulders. Breathing in, raise your head while depressing your spine. You may slide your arms forward as shown. Hold this position for as long as is comfortable. Breathe naturally.

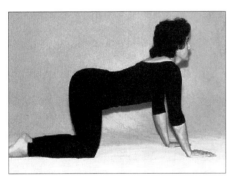 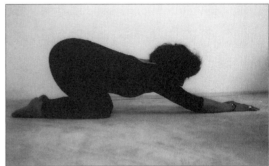

Breathing out, pull your stomach in and arch your back while lowering your head. Hold this position for as long as is comfortable. Breathe naturally. Repeat as often as you wish.

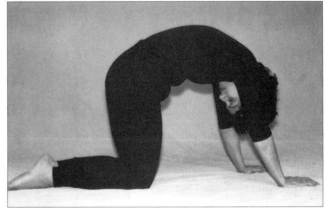

Benefits

Relaxes the arms, neck, shoulders, entire back, and abdominal area. Tones the reproductive system. Relieves menstrual and other cramps.

CAMEL (Ushtrasana)

A great pose for body conditioning, similar to that of weight lifting!

Practice A

Sit on your heels with your feet flat. Allow your arms to rest at your side.
Slowly move your arms one by one to the back, while arching your trunk
backwards and slightly lowering your head. Close your eyes and maintain
normal breathing. Hold this position for as long as is comfortable. Your
natural breathing becomes deeper due to the chest expansion.

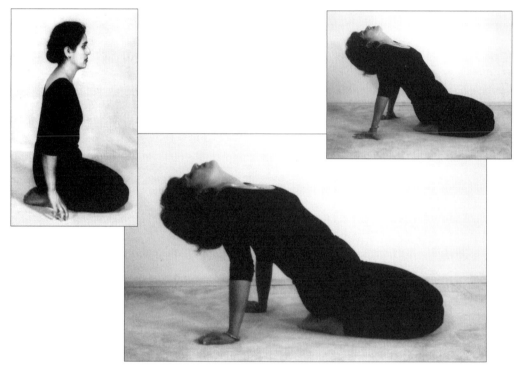

Precautions

Proceed to practice B, C, and D only after you have accomplished practice
A with ease and comfort. If you have carpal tunnel syndrome, you may
abstain from fully resting palms on the floor, as shown in the inset. Al-
ternatively you may make a fist and rest on it instead.

Practice B

Practice this pose as described in practice A, except, raise your hips as shown below.

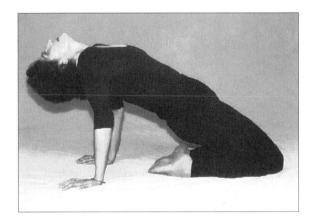

If your body allows, you may lift your hips further while moving your arms towards your body.

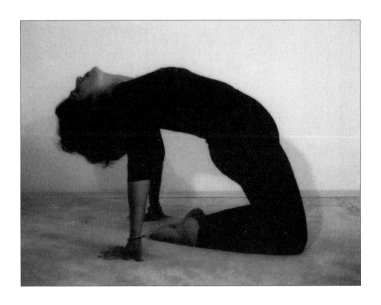

Practice C

Sit on your heels with your toes bent. Allow your arms to rest at your side. Slowly move your arms one by one to the back, while arching your trunk backwards and slightly lowering your head. Close your eyes and maintain normal breathing throughout. Hold the position for a comfortable length of time. Your natural breathing gets deeper due to the chest expansion.

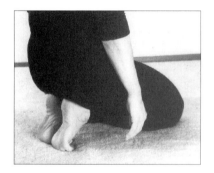

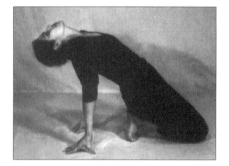

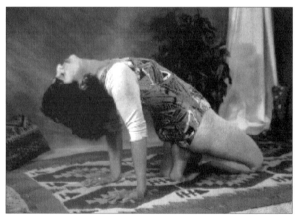

Practice D

Proceed with caution.

Sit on your heels or bent toes as in practice A and C. Stand on your knees with feet either flat or toes pointing down. Bend backwards and hold on to your heels as shown.

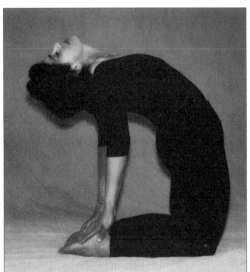
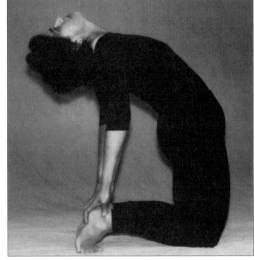

Benefits

Stretches the entire back, promoting spinal flexibility. Strengthens and tones the arms, shoulders, hips, and legs. Helps relieve tendinitis and carpal tunnel syndrome. Relaxes and strengthens the heart muscles. Exercises the lungs. Encourages deep breathing, which works as an excellent remedy for lung ailments such as colds, allergies, and asthma. Loosens stiff neck and shoulder muscles. Stretches and massages the facial muscles and skin as well as the neck. Helps normalize thyroid functioning.

SHOULDER STAND³ (Sarva Anga Asana)

A great pose with tremendous benefits for every part of the body!

Practice

Note: If you find it difficult to practice this posture, you may practice preliminary headstand instead.

Lie flat on your back, with your arms at your sides. Next, press your palms against the floor. Breathing out, slowly lift your trunk and legs while tightening your abdominal, hip, and leg muscles as shown on the next page.

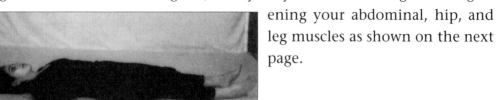

Beginners or people with a stiff back may stay in this position without raising the hips any further.

³ The name '*sarva*' means all and '*anga*' means parts or limbs. As the name implies, this is a great pose for every part of the body.

Beginners may raise their head and upper body in order to facilitate lifting the hips and trunk.

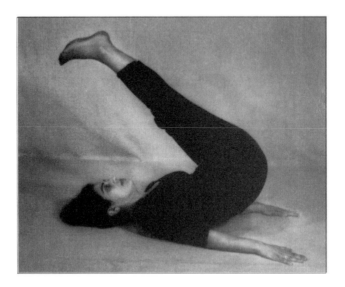

Support your hips with your hands as shown. Stay in the position for 30-60 seconds breathing naturally.

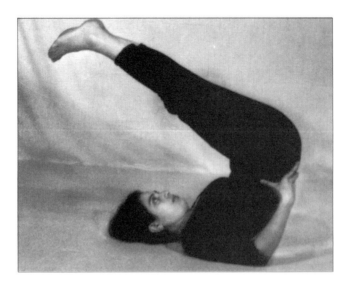

As your practice gets advanced, you may straighten your trunk and legs as much as possible, while lowering your palms for further support. Practice rectal contractions to intensify the benefits. Hold the position for as long as is comfortable while breathing naturally.

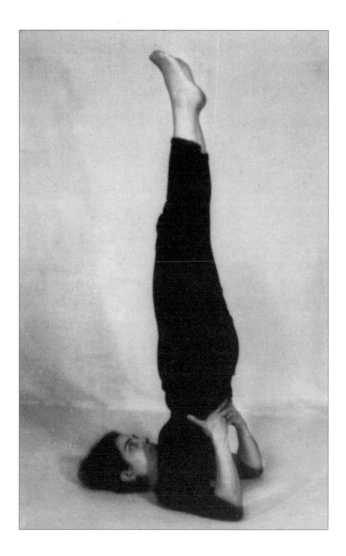

Slowly lower your legs and trunk while resting your arms on the floor.

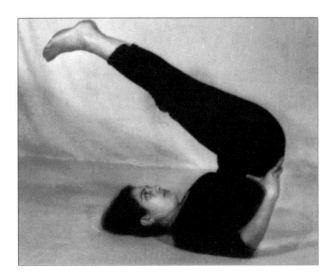

Remember to tighten abdominal, hip, and leg muscles as you lower your trunk and legs.

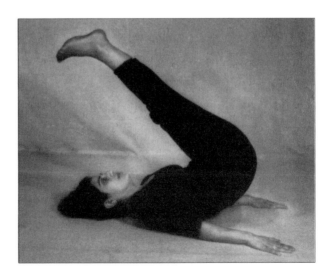

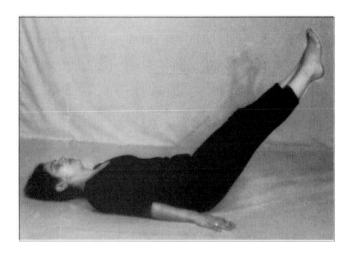

Relax completely before repeating this posture or attempting another.

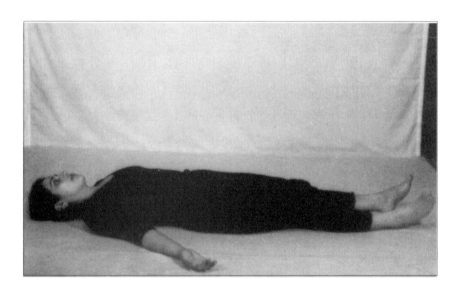

Variations

From the shoulder stand, slowly lower your left leg as much as possible. Stay in the position for 15-30 seconds while breathing naturally. Repeat the same movement with the right leg.

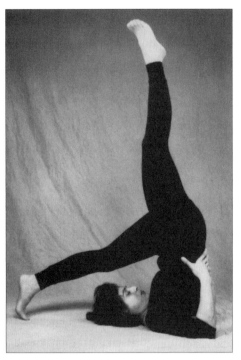

If you are able to sit in the lotus pose, try this variation.

Sit in the lotus position. Lie down. Follow the steps as in the shoulder stand.

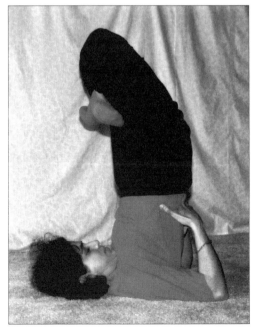

Benefits

Maintains general health and helps alleviate or prevent many ailments. Balances and regulates the activities of the endocrine system. Maintains and restores youthfulness by relaxing the internal glands and balancing the emotions and energy. Stimulates thyroid glands, normalizing the functioning of the thyroid (hypo or hyper); helps control, maintain, and properly distribute body weight. Helps alleviate headaches, improve eyesight, prevent hair loss, brings a glow to the face by increasing the supply of blood towards the head. Refreshes the mind by revitalizing brain cells. Relieves many lung ailments such as minor colds, allergy, asthma, and emphysema. Helps asthmatics overcome shallow breathing by encouraging diaphragmatic (abdominal) breathing. Relaxes the heart. Provides relief for varicose vein. Helps strengthen weak bladder and uterus by reversing the gravitational pull against the body. Provides an excellent therapy for people who are on their feet most of the time. When practiced with the rectal contractions, helps prevent prostrate cancer and other reproductive disorders.

PLOUGH (Halasana)

A great rejuvenator!

Practice

Note: You may either practice the plough separately or assume the plough position by lowering your legs directly after practicing the shoulder stand.

Lie flat on your back, with your arms at your side.

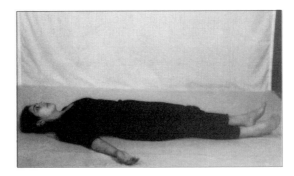

Breathing out, press your palms against the floor and slowly lift your trunk and legs, while tightening your abdominal, hip, and leg muscles.

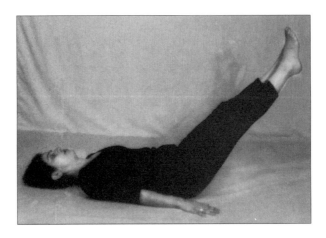

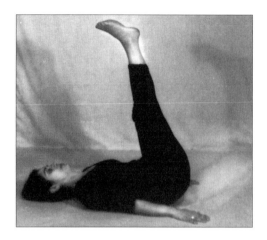

Lower your legs until they are parallel to the floor. Support your hips with your hands as shown. Breathe naturally in this position for 30-60 seconds.

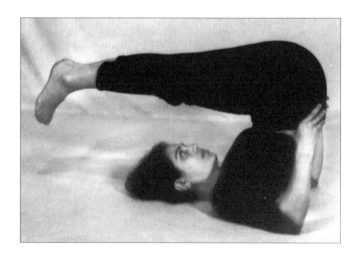

Be sure to pull your stomach in while breathing out as you lower your legs further. Maintain normal breathing. Stay in this position for as long as you are comfortable. Never use force or strain in order to attain this position.

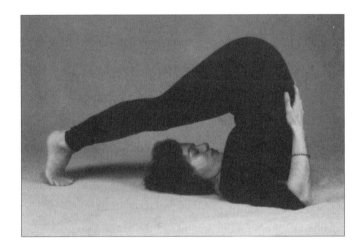

In the beginning, you may bend your legs at the knees. At this point, you may hold your back for support.

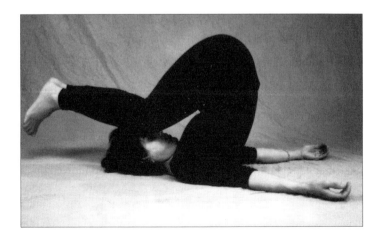

Slowly come out of the position as shown. Remember to tighten your abdominal, hip, and leg muscles as you lower your trunk.

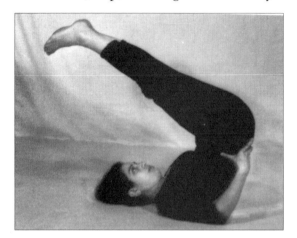

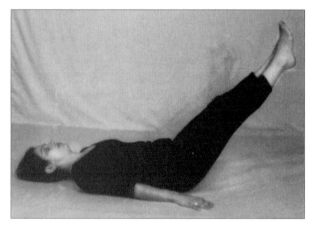

Relax completely before repeating the plough or attempting another posture.

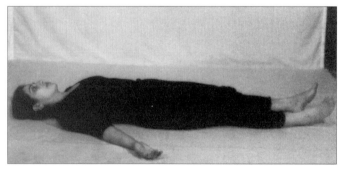

Variations

As you become comfortable with the plough, you may hold your toes either with your legs closer or apart as shown.

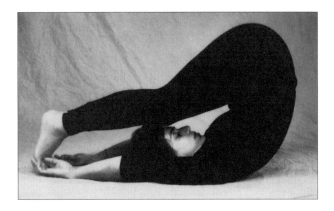

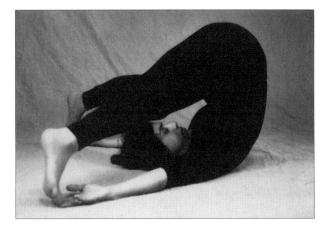

Benefits

Compliments all the benefits of the shoulder stand. Rejuvenates and revives the practitioner due to the excellent stretch of the spine and provides immediate relief for upper back and neck tension. Massages and tones the kidneys, liver, gall bladder, and other abdominal organs, improving their functions. Improves digestion. Provides relief for cramps and constipation. Helps alleviate and prevent diabetes by stimulating the pancreas.

COBRA (Bhujangasana)

A great physical tension reliever and energizer!

Practice

Lie on your stomach, with your palms resting below your shoulders and your chin resting on the floor.

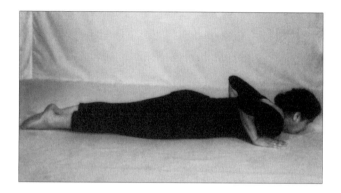

Breathing in, straighten you arms and lift your trunk. Hold the position for a comfortable length of time. Breathe naturally in the position. (With practice, your natural breath becomes deeper.) Breathing out, lower your trunk and head, resting your cheek on the floor, arms by your side.

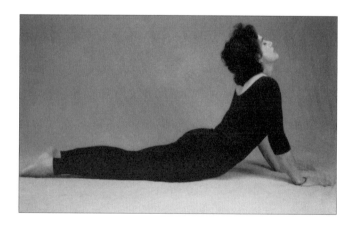

You may move your palms forward to ease the stretch. This is an easy position for beginners to attempt.

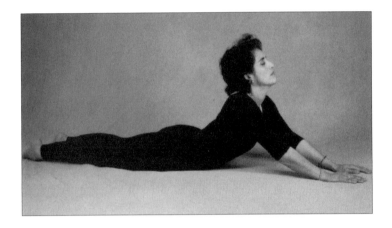

Variations

While in the cobra pose, raise your heels, bend your toes, and gently turn your head to the right. Stay in the position for 10-15 seconds. Repeat this while turning to the left. Note that your heels are raised with toes bent.

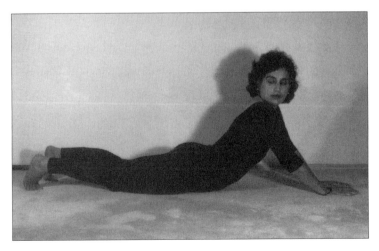

In the advanced stage, you may bend your legs as shown for additional benefits. You may further raise your torso as shown in the inset.

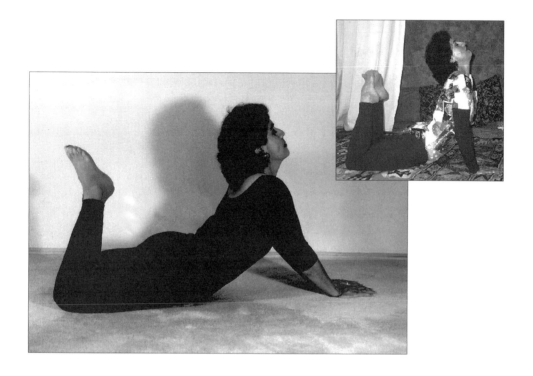

Benefits

Releases the vital energy from the base of the spine. Relieves back pain by gently stretching the vertebrae from the base of the spine to the neck. Strengthens arms, neck, shoulders, chest, abdominal muscles, and hips. Aids in relieving carpal tunnel syndrome by exercising the forearms, wrist joints, palms, and fingers. Stimulates the thyroid glands. Encourages deep respiration, which in turn strengthens the lungs and heart. Purifies the blood stream. Provides massaging action for the kidneys, thereby helping to prevent and reduce kidney stones.

PLANE

An easy stretch for the spine.

Practice

Lie flat on your stomach, arms by your side. Lift your arms and legs as high as possible while breathing naturally. You can also stretch your arms in front of you as shown.

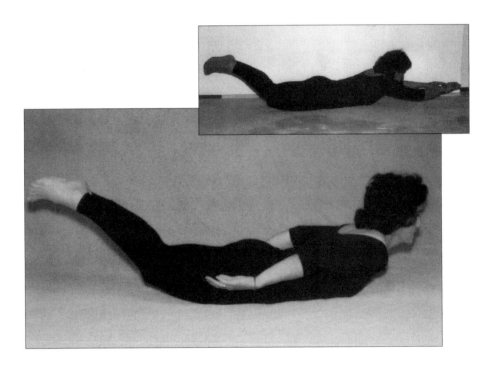

Benefits

Tones the spine, hips, abdomen, arms, and legs. Provides relief from backaches. Exercises the lungs and heart.

LOCUST (Shalabhasana)

An excellent pose for releasing vital energy from the base of the spine.

Practice A

Lie on your stomach, arms resting at your side and chin on the floor. Breathing naturally, slowly lift your legs as high as possible. Lift your arms slightly to balance the move. Stay in this position for 10-15 seconds. Come out of the position and rest your cheek and arms on the floor.

If you are unable to lift both legs simultaneously, you may try this variation by lifting one leg at a time.

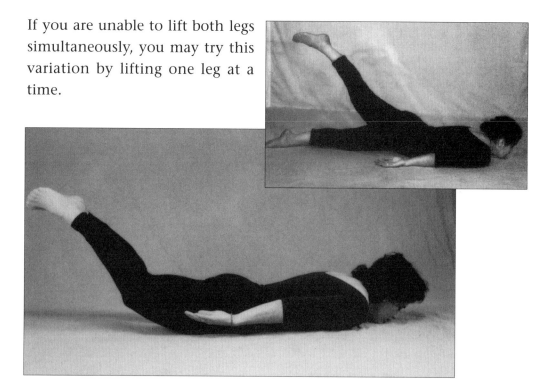

Practice B

Lie on your stomach, arms resting at your side and chin resting on the floor. Make tight fists and rest them below your hip joints or at your side. Breathing naturally, lift your legs while pressing your wrists against the floor. Stay in this position for 5-15 seconds. Do not strain in order to stay longer in this position, as it could cause tension for the heart. Come out of the position, relax your arms, and rest your cheek on the floor. Repeat if you wish.

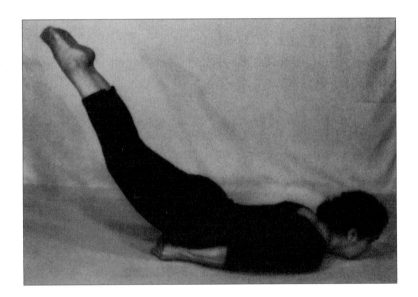

Benefits

Strengthens the base of the spine. Helps prevent slipped disc and other spinal injuries. Also, strengthens the legs, buttocks, hips, and sciatic nerves. Provides weight lifting effects for arm and wrist joints. Massages and tones pancreas, kidneys, liver, intestines, and reproductive organs. Helps strengthen the bladder. Helps prevent and alleviate prostrate, colon, and other cancers. Exercises the heart and lungs.

BOW (Dhanurasana)

A quick and great massage for the whole body!

Practice

Lie on your stomach, arms resting at your side and chin resting on the floor. Bend your legs at the knees and hold your ankles. Try to keep your arms straight.

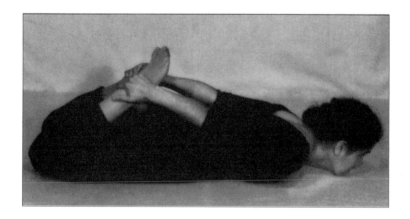

Slowly raise your head and knees from the floor without bending your arms. Hold this position while breathing naturally for a comfortable duration.

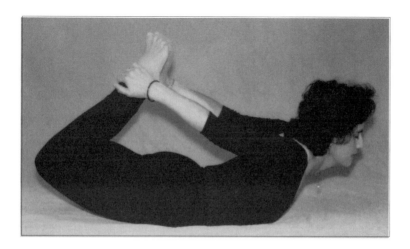

As you become comfortable, you may attempt to stretch up further by raising your knees and chest. Come out of the position, resting your cheek, arms, and legs on the floor.

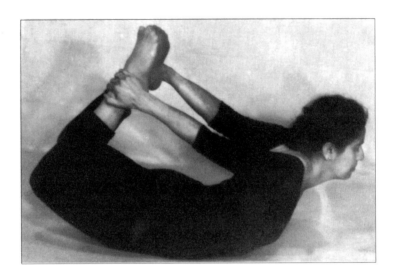

Benefits

Stretches and massages the entire body. Stimulates the pancreas, kidney, and liver, regulating their functions. Regulates cortisone secretion by stimulating the adrenal gland, which is also an aid for rheumatic pain. Because the bow is a combination of the cobra and locust, it also provides all the benefits of these poses.

PRELIMINARY LEG PULL (Paschimottanasana)

A great muscular tension reliever!

Practice

Sit on the floor with your legs extended and your hands resting on your legs. Breathing in deeply, lift your arms above your head.

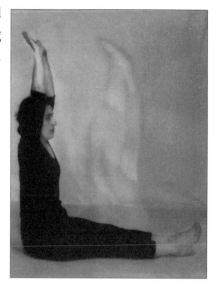

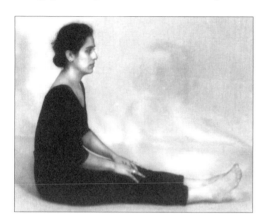

Breathing out, pulling your stomach in, bend forward while sliding your hands on your legs. Hold your legs comfortably and breathe naturally in the position for 15-30 seconds.

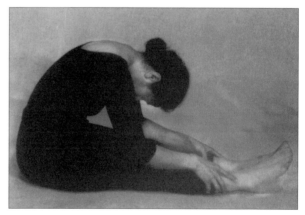

Once you are very comfortable, stretch further as you breathe out. You may further reach out to hold your feet or toes.

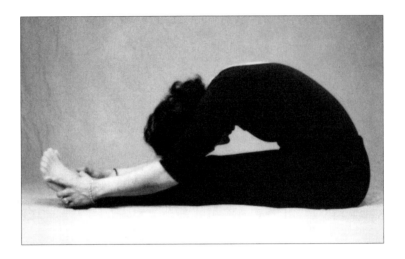

Benefits

Gently stretches and tones the entire spine. Eases back pain. Improves digestion. Firms the abdominal muscles. Relieves menstrual or other cramps. Helps prevent and alleviate diabetes, ulcers, fibroid growths, colon cancer, and other stress-related abdominal aliments. Stretches and strengthens the sciatic nerves, hamstrings, and knees. The increased stretch and improved blood circulation throughout the body provide tremendous relief from arthritic pains.

FISH (Matsyasana)

A great relief for lung ailments!

Practice

Sit on your heels, with your arms by your side.

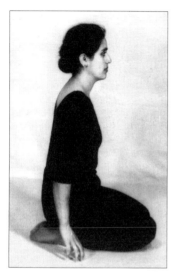

Leaning back, rest your palms behind you, with your fingers facing forward.

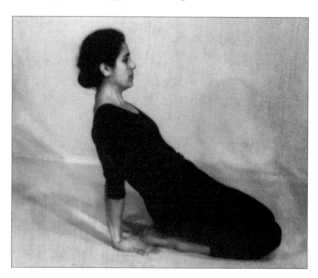

Rest on your elbows one at a time.

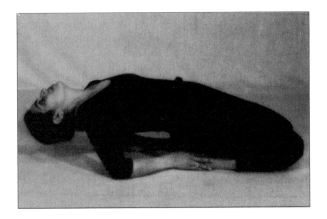

As you slide your arms forward, arch your back and rest the crown of your head on the floor. Hold the position while breathing normally for 15-30 seconds.

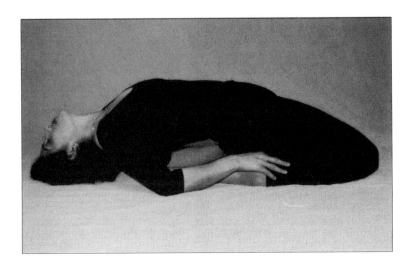

Once you are comfortable, you may rest your arms on your abdomen while increasing the arch of your back. Breathe naturally in the position for 30-60 seconds. (When you are comfortable in this position, your breath naturally becomes deeper.)

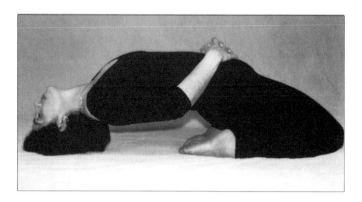

To come out of the pose, support yourself with your elbows, rest the nape of the neck, roll to the side, and then lift yourself up. You can also come out by sitting up straight using your arms for support.

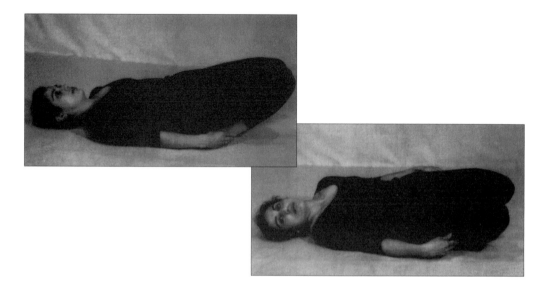

Variation

This variation is an easy alternative for beginners or for those who are unable to do the complete fish pose.

Lie flat on your back with your legs bent. Raise your hips and place your hands under them, palms facing the floor. Now straighten your legs, arch your back, and rest the top of your head on the floor. Hold this position for 10-30 seconds while breathing normally. Come out of the pose by bringing your arms out and rest them by your side while resting the nape of your neck on the floor.

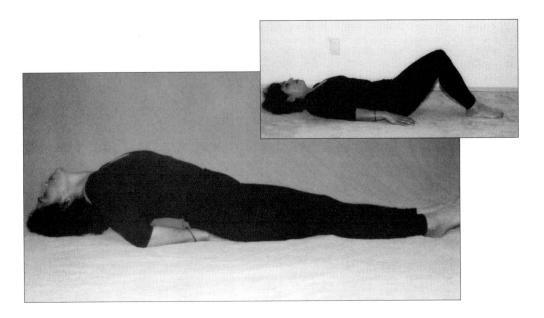

Benefits

Stretches and strengthens the spine, neck, abdomen, and chest muscles. Massages the upper back, neck, and facial muscles. Stimulates the thyroid glands. Encourages deep breathing and exercises the chest muscles; provides immediate relief from wheezing, asthmatic symptoms, and other respiratory ailments; helps alleviate heart ailments and prevent breast cancer.

PSYCHIC UNION POSE (Yoga Mudra)

A quick way to get in touch with your inner self.

Practice

Sit in the easy, half, or full lotus. You may either hold your wrist or interlock your fingers behind you.

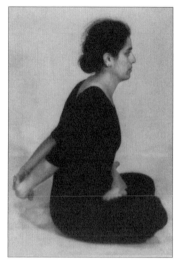

Breathe in deeply. Breathing out, pull your stomach in and bend forward as much as you can. Breathe naturally in this position for 30-60 seconds. Come out of the position as you breathe in.

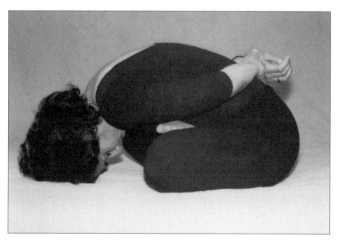

Variations

You could either straighten your arms behind you or stretch your arms in front of you while sitting in the easy lotus position, as shown. Alternately, you may rest your arms by your side as in the turtle pose.

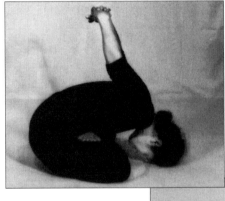

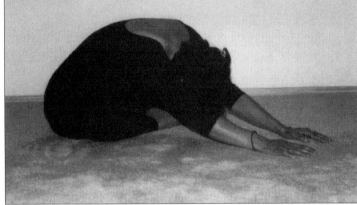

Benefits

Provides a gentle and soothing stretch for the spine and hips. Massages the hips and abdominal area. Releases the tension from the upper back and chest muscles. Provides immediate mental relaxation; increases self awareness.

ALTERNATE LEG PULL (Janu Sirshasana)

A great energy balancer!

Practice

Sit with your left leg extended and your right leg bent at the knee so your foot rests beside your left thigh.

As you breathe in, lift your arms straight up. Breathing out, bend toward your outstretched leg and stretch forward as much as you can. Breathe naturally. Remain in the position for 15-30 seconds. Breathing in, come out of the posture and return to the sitting position. Repeat this procedure with the right leg extended.

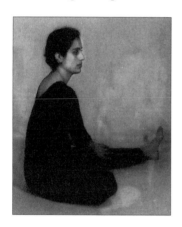
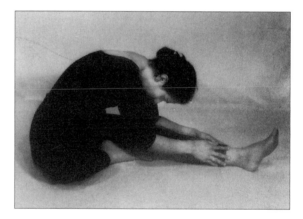

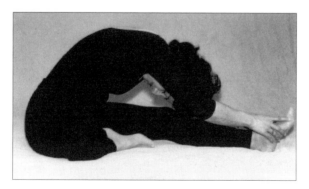

Variation

As your practice advances, you may rest your right foot on your left thigh and try to hold your foot or toes with both hands.

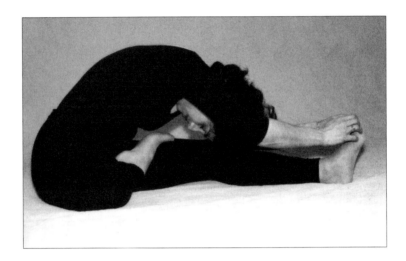

Benefits

Stretches and relaxes the arms, neck, upper back, spine, hamstrings, sciatic nerves, and both sides of the hips. Massages the kidneys. Trims the waistline and strengthens the abdominal area.

SPINAL TWIST (Vakrasana)

A great spine conditioner!

Practice

Sit with your legs extended. Cross your right leg over your left and rest your right foot or heel on the floor. Breathing out, move your left arm over your right leg and hold your left leg. You may rest your arm in various positions as shown in the insets. From your waist upwards, twist your body to you right, while placing your right arm behind you. With your palm or fingers resting on the floor, try looking to your right, twisting as much as you can. Throughout this pose, your buttocks should be fully resting on the floor. Remain upright and do not lean backward or sideways. Hold the position for 15-30 seconds while breathing naturally. Breathing in, release the twist and return to the sitting position. Repeat this stretch on the other side by reversing the positions of your legs and arms as shown on the next page.

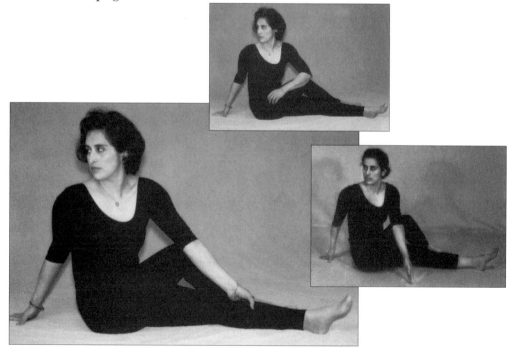

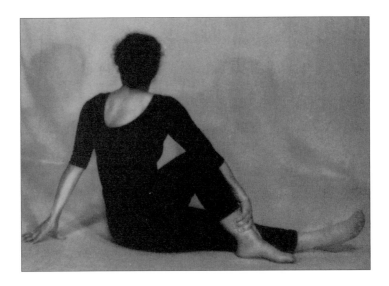

You may rest the back of your hand against the side of your waist as shown.

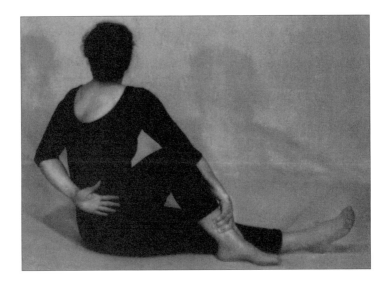

Variation

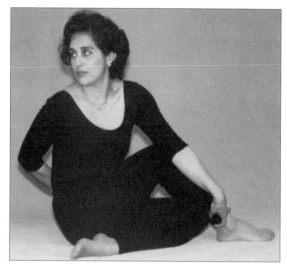

Instead of extending the leg, you may bend it toward the opposite hip.

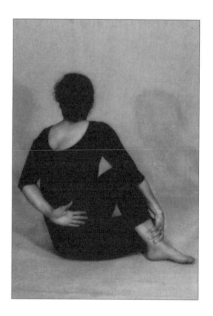

Benefits

Provides a great twist for the spine, arms, upper back, neck, and shoulders. Massages the abdominal area, regulating the activities of the pancreas, digestive system, kidneys, liver, and spleen. Eliminates constipation. Provides relief for rheumatic and arthritic pain. Trims the waistline. Exercises the lungs and relaxes the heart muscles.

ROUTINES[4]

Here is a summary of different yoga routines. You may choose from either the Beginner/Intermediate or the Advanced routines based on your level of experience. Depending on the amount of time available, you may practice any one of the listed routines.

BEGINNER/INTERMEDIATE ROUTINES

Detailed Routine

Ankle rotation

Butterfly

Churning the mill

Leg lock

Cycling

Neck movements

Shoulder socket rotation

Triangle stretch

Double angle

Salutation to the sun (*1 round*)

Corpse relaxation

Pose of the moon

Cat

Camel (*practice A or B*)

Shoulder stand

Plough

Cobra

Preliminary leg pull

Spinal twist

Two leg lock

Corpse relaxation

Quick Routine 1

Ankle rotation

Leg lock

Lying twist

Cat

Mountain pose

Cobra

Turtle pose or pose of the moon

Spinal twist

Corpse relaxation

Quick Routine 2

Toe and back stretch

One leg stretch

Feet and palm stretch

Salutation to the Sun (*2 rounds*)

Corpse relaxation

[4] For additional routines, refer to Appendix C.

ADVANCED ROUTINES

DETAILED ROUTINE

Leg lock

Lying twist

Sit-ups

One leg stretch

Warrior pose

Toe and back stretch

Arm and leg stretch

Salutation to the sun (*2 rounds*)

Corpse relaxation

Shoulder stand

Plough

Fish or camel

Psychic union or pose of the moon

Cobra

Locust

Bow

Preliminary leg pull

Alternate leg pull

Spinal twist

Two leg lock

Corpse relaxation

QUICK ROUTINE 1

Leg lock

Lying twist

Shoulder stand

Plough

Camel

Turtle or bowing pose

Spinal twist

Corpse relaxation

QUICK ROUTINE 2

Salutation to the sun (*3 rounds*)

(*Stay in steps 3, 4, 7, 8 and 9 for about 30 seconds in the final round. Breathe naturally while holding these positions.*)

Corpse relaxation

Notes:

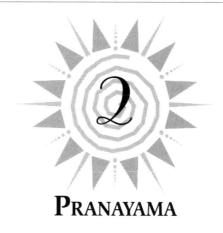

PRANAYAMA

"Prana is a wonderful healing energy that is free and always available!"

Prana is referred to as the "universal life energy" because it is the life force or cosmic energy that pervades all things. In nature, prana can be seen in the way plants grow, in the migrations and activities of animals, in the passing of the seasons, and even in the geological evolution of the mountains and landscape around us. In our lives, prana is our vital energy, our life force. We absorb prana from the food we eat, the water we drink, the air we breathe, and the other energies around us. In turn, we expend prana in our life activities by moving, thinking, talking, digesting food, and performing other life functions. When sufficient prana is present in the body, we experience radiant health and general well-being. Our thoughts, movements, and internal body functions are in balance and serve our higher purpose. When insufficient prana is in the body, we experience stress, lack of motivation, and fatigue. We may feel rundown and depressed. The ancient yogis used the regular practice of pranayama techniques to absorb an abundance of prana and store the excess prana in the body, like a battery stores electricity. People with an abundance of prana are noticeably more energetic. They radiate energy and vitality to those around them. At the higher levels of practice, this abundance of prana can be utilized to help others heal, maintain our own health and well-being, raise our consciousness to higher levels, and uplift our spirituality. The practice of pranayama is the technique of balancing and restoring pranic energy through controlled breathing.

Our breath is the basic, external form of prana in our lives. As we breathe in and out, we experience the ebb and flow of life energy. However, as we learn to breathe more consciously, we can extend the power of prana beyond mere breath. Yoga asanas prepare the body by strengthening and clearing the pranic channels. Pranayama further helps cleanse and purify the pranic channels. When the pranic channels are strong and clear, pranayama can be practiced to direct the prana to the areas in need to release physical and emotional tension. When the body and mind are in a relaxed state, positive and energetic feelings come forth naturally even in difficult circumstances.

On the physical level, pranayama (controlled, conscious breathing) promotes the intake of oxygen which helps purify the blood and expel bodily toxins, such as carbon dioxide. It also improves the nervous and immune systems, and boosts stamina and endurance. The expansion and compression of the abdominal area during pranayama provide a gentle massage for the digestive and reproductive systems, and healing benefits to the internal organs, such as kidney, liver, and bladder. Similarly, the chest expansion and compression during pranayama help normalize cholesterol, triglyceride levels, clear blockages in the coronary arteries, and relieve stress-related symptoms, such as hypertension, high or low blood pressure, insomnia, headache, anxiety, nervousness, and irritability. Pranayama also helps alleviate chronic colds, asthma, sinus congestion, allergies, emphysema, snoring, and other lung ailments. In the advanced practice, pranayama can also be used as an effective treatment to help ease severe pain and heal conditions such as cancer and tumors.

Joan Arnest describes her use of yoga and pranayama to overcome chronic sinus infections and chest ailments. "Each Spring and Fall, I counted on getting a sinus infection. As others happily enjoyed the buds and blossoms of the seasons, I would start to sniffle, sneeze, and drip until my sinuses swelled and my head throbbed. I would get very ill. As I got older, these infections spread to my chest. Chest colds began turning into chronic bronchitis and the beginnings of asthma. It was at this time that I started taking yoga classes from Vasanthi. My goals were to stay flexible, help my muscles and bones stay strong, and hopefully learn to relax through meditation. I had no idea yoga and pranayama would help with my sinus and chest problems. Part of every yoga session with Vasanthi is spent doing pranayama exercises, such as alternate nostril breathing, deep breathing, rhythmic breathing, bellows breath, sniffing, and more. I was a good student and practiced some at home, especially the alternate nostril breathing done with a chin lock. Slowly as the months went by my head and chest were cleared up. I had only one or two mild sinus infections, but my air passageways were no longer clogged. I can very happily say that I have not had any chest ailments since I began practicing yoga regularly. It has been a wonderful blessing, and I feel truly thankful."

On the mental or emotional level, pranayama helps you gain control over your mind and emotions, and acts as a tonic to mental and emotional fatigue. It induces calmness and tranquility, providing immediate relief from daily stress. It also helps improve concentration, will power, and tolerance. When practiced after yoga asanas, pranayama techniques naturally lead to a deep and peaceful meditation. Pranayama helps draw prana into the body and directs the prana to where it is most needed. The flow and balance of prana relaxes and heals the body, naturally leading to deeper consciousness and spirituality.

Srinu Sista, a software engineer, discovered that yoga and pranayama helped him overcome fatigue and find tranquility. "In the beginning of my practice, I would be so tired after all the asanas that I would just fall asleep and to the chagrin and/or amusement of the rest of the class, I would snore loudly and perhaps keep every one else awake. As I progressed in the classes, I had more energy and was able to do the asanas more efficiently without getting tired. The result was that the concluding meditation was more effective. (I fell asleep less often and, when I did fall asleep, the class noticed I no longer snored.) Instead of falling asleep, I would quietly rest and my mind would be cleansed of all negative thoughts of the whole week. I would find myself content with my own well-being and a sense of peace and tranquility would fill me. Afterward, I was more refreshed and ready to take on my next challenge."

In more practical ways, the techniques of pranayama can also be used to complement vigorous activities, such as swimming, running, dancing, and singing. Proper breathing enhances enjoyment and performance.

Hema Sista, an engineer and Carnatic classical singer, practices yoga and pranayama to ease her allergies and enhance her singing. "I first started yoga because as a vocalist, I wanted to increase my lung power and keep my voice in shape. My voice was getting hoarse. During a visit to the allergist, I was informed that I was a 'walking time bomb', badly in need of allergy shots, since I was allergic to about 90% of the allergens tested! Last year, I completely lost my voice for about three months. The ENT specialist prescribed anti-allergy medication, asking me to take it twice a day. Being a believer in holistic medicine, I was averse to taking any sort of medication. I spoke to Vasanthi, and she suggested several asanas and pranayama which I have been practicing, including one to keep my sinuses clear. I have since not had any episodes of losing my voice. In addition, I do not take any allergy medications, nor do I take allergy shots. I do not suffer from the symptoms of allergy that I have had for so many years before I started yoga."

Best of all, pranayama can be practiced by anyone, regardless of age or physical condition. Pranayama techniques are very flexible and can be practiced anytime of the day and anywhere that is convenient. Although they are generally practiced sitting with the back straight, these techniques can also be practiced standing in front of an open window or door, outdoors, at work, or anywhere you can consciously focus on your breath. Because access to clear air is a requirement, be sure to practice when the air is clear and not polluted. For example, if you live in an urban city, be careful not to practice pranayama close to traffic fumes or industrial smog. Breathing contaminated air can result in serious respiratory problems.

Once the yogic breathing or pranayama techniques are regularly practiced, their power and benefit will become apparent to you. Their versatility will also be appealing as you find ways and places to practice and use them throughout the day. After you experience how each one affects your body, you can choose the appropriate ones for your specific situations. For example, when you feel anxious and want to balance your emotions, practice a few rounds of alternate nostril breathing or complete breathing. In addition to relieving anxiety and discomfort, you can also expand the practice of alternate nostril breathing or complete breathing to uplift your spirituality and develop higher consciousness. This practice will further awaken the kundalini energy[1] stored near the base of your spine.

When you feel sluggish and want to energize yourself, practice a few rounds of bellows breath. You will soon feel refreshed and balanced. You can also practice bellows breath when you feel constipated, have abdominal cramps, or just want to tone the abdominal area.

Premlata Majmundar, a retired teacher and senior yoga student, practices bellows breath to strengthen her abdominal area and to feel refreshed. "When I practice bellows breath in the morning, I feel very good and energetic. This practice also helps strengthen my stomach."

---

[1] For information on awakening the kundalini energy, refer to the chapter on meditation.

The table below briefly lists the benefits of pranayama techniques.

Pranayama Techniques	Benefits
• Simple breathing	Warm-up technique.
• Complete breathing	Purifies and strengthens the breathing channels.
• Double breath	Relieves tension.
• Sniffing A & B	Relaxes the mind and improves concentration.
• Chin lock A & B	Releases sinus pressure.
• Rectal contraction	Retains pranic energy.
• Alternate nostril breathing	Purifies breathing channels and balances emotions.
• Rhythmic breathing	Strengthens the lungs and heart.
• Bellows breath	Purifies the lungs and massages the abdominal area.
• Panting breath	Restores energy.
• Lion breath	Exercises the lungs. Relieves chest congestion. Soothes the throat. Stretches facial and eye muscles.
• Cooling breath	Relaxes the nervous system. Cools the whole body.
• Energy renewing breath	Stimulates the pressure points around the neck, relaxing the whole system.
• Bee sounding breath	Relieves mental fatigue.
• Om chanting	Vibrates the lungs. Relaxes the body and mind.
• Corpse relaxation	Relaxes the body, mind, and emotions.

You may practice the techniques as they are listed or as shown at the end of this chapter. Be sure to always start your regular practice with simple breathing and continue with the techniques that are best for you. Simple breathing eases your system and serves as a warm-up preceding other techniques. If you are practicing for specific ailments, increase the practicing time or rounds.

THINGS TO KNOW BEFORE PRACTICING PRANAYAMA

- It is best to practice pranayama in the morning when the air is clear and fresh. However, if morning practice is not possible, practice in the evening or anytime the air is clean and free of pollution. Be sure to practice in a well-ventilated area.

- Ensure that you are seated comfortably in the lotus, half-lotus, easy lotus position, or in a chair. If any of these positions are un-comfortable, you may sit on a cushion, or lean against a wall or a piece of furniture to support your back. However, you can also lie down on the floor or bed if your physical condition does not enable you to sit up.

- To experience the benefits, it is not necessary to practice all the pranayama techniques in a continuous sequence. Practice those that are comfortable for you and suit your situation. Also, do not post-pone your practice merely because there isn't sufficient time for all the techniques you want to practice. You may adopt different techniques and combinations to suit your needs and situation. Even as little as 2-10 minutes of practice per day is beneficial. When all else fails, find a few moments to check your breathing rhythm and breathe consciously. This alone can hold you over until there is enough time to practice the techniques.

- Most pranayama techniques are practiced breathing through the nostrils. The lion and cooling breath techniques are exceptions that require breathing through the mouth.

- For general health, practice the techniques for 3-5 rounds. For specific ailments, you may increase the number of repetitions. Remember to rest for about 10-15 seconds between pranayama techniques.

- Be aware that several pranayamas involve stomach compression and are best practiced on an empty stomach. Do not use strain to hold or lengthen your breath.

- If you have a sinus, respiratory, or heart ailment, you may experience dizziness or shortness of breath during practice. When this occurs, immediately stop the practice and return to your normal breathing until the dizziness or shortness of breath eases. With practice, the dizziness and shortness of breath will gradually diminish and disap-pear.

PRANAYAMA TECHNIQUES

These are the positions that are generally adopted for practicing pranayama. Or you may adopt any position that suits your body.

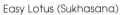
Easy Lotus (Sukhasana)

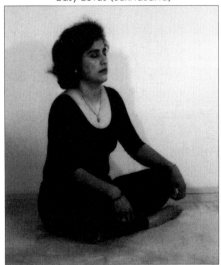

Half Lotus (Siddhasana)

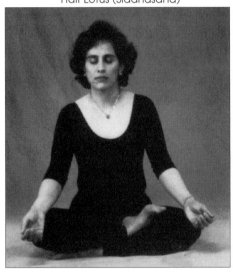

Full Lotus (Padmasana)

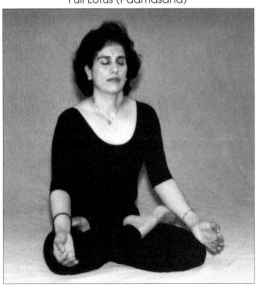

Easy Lotus on a cushion

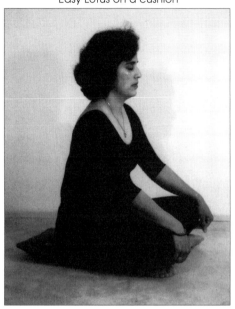

Sitting on heels (Vajrasana)

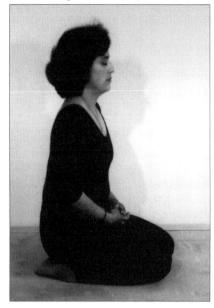

Sitting in a chair

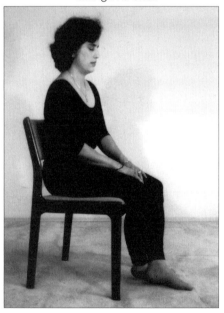

SIMPLE BREATHING

Simple or natural breathing is our involuntary breathing. It is the foundation for all the other breathing techniques and a key to happiness.

Practice

Sit comfortably with your back straight. Close your eyes. Focus your awareness on your breath. Feel your breath flow in and out through your nostrils. Do not change the breathing pattern. Do not strain or use force. Let yourself breathe naturally. As you breathe, ensure that your chest and stomach are involved in each breath. Observe how your stomach and chest muscles expand and compress as you breathe in and out. Remain focused on your breath for about a minute (15-30 breaths) or until your breath becomes steady and relaxed. Once breath awareness[2] is established, you will be able to consciously apply it in your postures, meditation, and daily life.

Benefits

Develops breath awareness. Eases emotional and mental stress. Prepares your mind, body, and breath for other pranayama exercises by improving concentration.

[2] Conscious breathing involves focusing your awareness on the flow of your breath. It does not require you to breathe deeply. Just direct your total attention to your natural breath.

COMPLETE BREATHING

A natural extension of simple breathing.

Practice

Sit comfortably with your back straight. Close your eyes. Focus your awareness on your natural breath. Gently prolong the exhalation while pulling your stomach in as much as possible. As you breathe in, let your compressed stomach come up naturally[3] and breathe upward while expanding the chest sideways. Breathe out from the chest to the stomach while pulling the stomach in as slowly as you can. Good complete breathing always starts with good exhalation. Notice how the inhalation improves after good exhalation. Do this procedure gently and slowly like a smooth wave flowing up from the stomach to the chest as you breathe in and flowing down from the chest to the stomach as you breathe out. Never allow your stomach to jerk as you breathe. Notice that after a few deep breaths, your breathing becomes smoother and deeper. Practice for about 15 breaths or 1-2 minutes. Rest for about 10-15 seconds before you start another pranayama.

Benefits

Eases insomnia, anxiety, nervousness, restlessness, hypertension, and other symptoms related to stress. Purifies and strengthens the breathing channels and lungs. Helps clear any blockages in the coronary arteries. Alleviates any lung ailments. Energizes and refreshes your body and mind. Strengthens and stimulates the abdominal area. Tones the kidneys, liver, bladder, and reproductive systems. Prevents and heals abdominal ailments – cramps, constipation, and any internal and external growths such as tumors and cancers. Aids in weight loss and weight maintenance. Improves digestion, stamina, endurance, tolerance, and the immune system.

---

[3] Make sure not to expand your stomach more than normal. Excessive expansion can restrict the flow of air to the upper chest.

DOUBLE BREATH

A quick tension reliever.

Practice

Stand, sit, or lie on your back with arms by your side. You may close your eyes if you wish. Breathe out deeply. After breathing out, take a short breath in, followed by a long, deep breath. Holding the breath, tense the whole body while making a fist and stretching your arms out. Hold the position for about 10 seconds. Release the tension as you breathe out. Repeat as often as you wish.

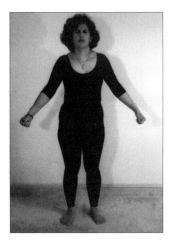
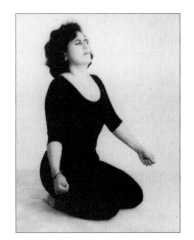

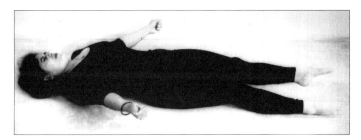

Benefits

Removes mental stress and physical tension. Provides quick and easy relaxation. Revitalizes each and every cell in your body by improving the circulation of prana.

SNIFFING (Viloma)

A great tranquilizer!

STEP A

Practice

Sit comfortably with your back straight. Close your eyes. Slowly breathe in using short, brisk inhalations, pausing in between them and filling the lungs moderately. Hold the breath for as long as is comfortable. Then, slowly breathe out, while gently pulling in your stomach as much as possible. Practice 2-3 rounds. Rest for a few moments before proceeding to the next step.

STEP B

Practice

Breathe in deeply, filling the lungs moderately. Hold your breath for a few seconds. Slowly breathe out in short, brisk exhalations, pausing between them. Keep doing this until your stomach is completely pulled in. Practice this technique for 2-3 rounds.

Benefits

Strengthens the lungs, bringing feelings of ease and lightness to the body and mind. Revitalizes each and every cell by improving the circulation of prana.

CHIN LOCK A and B (Jalandara Bandha)

An effective sinus congestion reliever.

Practice A[4]

Sit comfortably with your back straight and palms on your knees. Breathe in comfortably and hold your breath. Slowly lower your head and straighten your arms as you lift your shoulders so your chin rests on your chest. Hold this position for as long as is comfortable. Lower your shoulders as you raise your head. Be sure to breathe out only after raising your head. Repeat as often as you like.

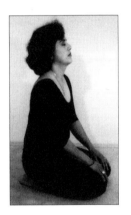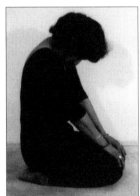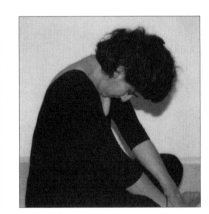

Practice B

Breathe in and out slowly and hold your breath out. Lower your head so your chin rests on your chest. Hold this position for as long as is comfortable. Be sure to breathe in after you lower the shoulders and raise your head up. Repeat as often as you wish.

Benefits

Improves concentration by stimulating the neck and concentration center. Releases any sinus pressure. Stimulates the thyroid glands.

---

[4] Chin lock A is an excellent technique to combine with alternate nostril breathing.

RECTAL CONTRACTION[5] (Moolabandha)

Helps retain vital energy.

Practice

Note: This technique can be included in any pranayama technique that involves holding the breath.

Breathe in and hold your breath. While holding your breath, tighten your rectal muscles, pulling them in as much as possible. Hold this position for as long as is comfortable. Release your rectal contraction and then breathe out.

When practicing chin lock and combining the chin lock in the alternate nostril breathing, practice rectal contraction after resting the chin on the chest. Release the contraction before you lift your chin up.

Benefits

Retains the vital energy. Helps awaken the kundalini energy hidden just below the base of the spine (mooladhara chakra). Aids in preventing and alleviating hemorrhoids and prostate cancer. Strengthens the bladder, pelvic area, reproductive system as well as the related muscles and organs.

---

[5] This can also be practiced as you breathe naturally in any position (sitting, standing, lying down) to strengthen the rectal, bladder, and other connected muscles.

ALTERNATE NOSTRIL BREATHING A, B, C, D (Nadi Shuddhi)

The most effective pranayama practice for cleansing and purifying the breathing channels!

Practice A (Natural Breathing)

Note: You may practice any one or all of the steps from A to D. When practicing all the steps, it is not necessary to rest in between.

Sit comfortably with your back straight. Close your eyes. Rest the index and middle fingers of your right hand on your eyebrow center. Close your right nostril with your thumb. Left-handed people need to switch the thumb and ring finger. Breathe in moderately through your left nostril and close it with your ring finger.

Open your right nostril and breathe out gently as shown on the next page. Breathe in through the right nostril and close your nostril. Open your left nostril and breathe out. This is one round. Breathe in through your left nostril to start the next round. Practice 3-5 rounds.

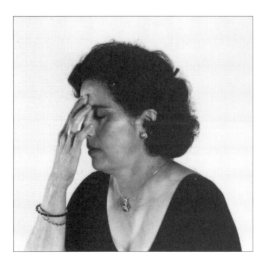
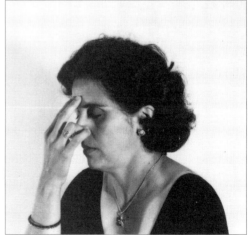

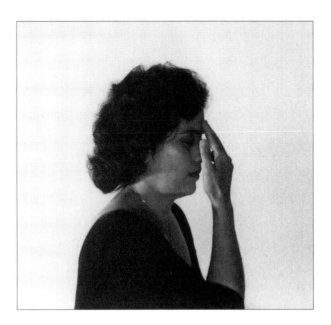

If you find that one of your nostrils is not fully clear, keep breathing gently and you will find that the blockage may slowly clear up. If it does not clear up, raise the arm opposite to your blocked nostril, press the armpit and lower your arm as shown. Hold the position until your nostril is clear.

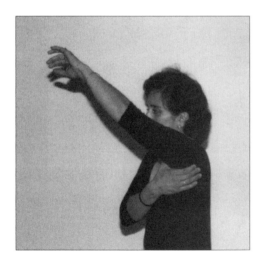 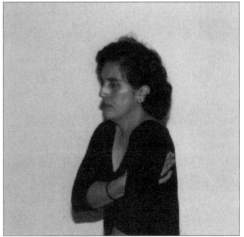

Practice B (Breath Retention)

Note: People with high blood pressure and/or heart problems are advised not to practice breath retention with strain in steps B, C, and D.

This technique is similar to Practice A except that you hold the inhaled breath for a moment. After you breathe in through your left nostril, close the nostril and hold your breath for a moment. (While holding your breath, you may also practice rectal contraction. Release the contraction before breathing out.) Open your right nostril and breathe out. Breathe in through your right nostril and close the nostril and hold your breath for a moment. (Repeat the rectal contraction.) Open your left nostril and breathe out. This is one round. For additional benefits, you may gradually increase the duration of the breath retention. Repeat 2-3 times. Rest briefly before moving on to the next practice.

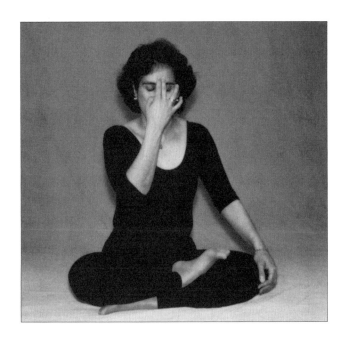

Practice C (Slow and Deep Breathing)

This is the same technique as Practice B except that this is with deep breathing. Breathe in slowly and deeply through the left nostril and close the nostril. Hold your breath as long as you can without strain. Open the right nostril and breathe out slowly and deeply. Breathe in deeply through your right nostril and hold your breath, and breathe out slowly through the left nostril.

It is very natural to feel like opening your mouth as you practice this breathing. This indicates your breathing channels are being cleansed. If this occurs, practice deep breathing a couple of times before proceeding with this practice.

Practice D (Chin Lock and Rectal Contraction)

This technique is similar to Practice C except that you include the chin lock and rectal contraction after holding your breath. Breathe in through the left nostril and hold your breath. Holding your breath, lower your head to practice the chin lock and the rectal contraction. Release the contraction before

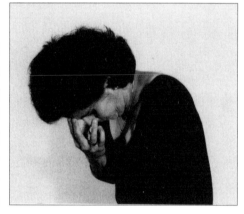

you raise your head. With your face up, open your right nostril and breathe out. Breathe in through your right nostril, hold your breath and practice the chin lock and the rectal contraction. Release the contraction and with your face up, open your left nostril and breathe out. This is one round. For additional benefits, you can gradually increase the duration of your breath retention.

Benefits

Induces calmness and tranquility; helps alleviate mental and emotional tension. Highly effective for relieving insomnia, hypertension, depression, anger, and nervousness. Clears the breathing channels and pranic passages of any blockages. Helps relieve lung ailments, such as allergy, asthma, and chronic cold. Helps clear fat deposits in the coronary arteries. Balances the flow of prana in the sympathetic and parasympathetic nerves (ida and pingala). When practiced with chinlock and rectal contractions, it serves as the most important preparation for advanced meditation.

RHYTHMIC BREATHING (Samavritti)

A great relaxation for the mind.

Practice

Sit comfortably with your back straight. Breathe in and hold your breath. Breathe out and hold your breath out. This is one round. Repeat these four steps rhythmically and evenly for 3-5 rounds. This technique is very effective when practiced without any strain. Refer to Chapter 3 on meditation for more information about counting and chanting during this practice.

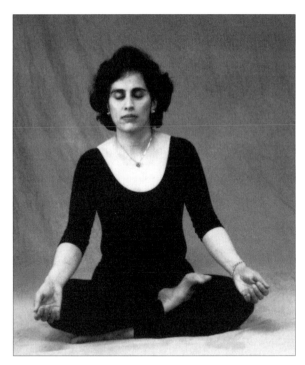

Benefits

Strengthens the lungs, relaxes the heart, and brings immediate relaxation to the mind. Improves concentration and prepares the mind for meditation. Provides an easy technique to relieve insomnia.

BELLOWS BREATH (Kapalabhati)

Instant Energizer!

Practice

Note: People with high blood pressure and/or heart problems are advised to practice this technique at a slower tempo.

Assume a comfortable sitting position with your back straight. Breathe in deeply. Breathe out forcefully while contracting the stomach muscles quickly and rhythmically, pushing them toward the spine and relaxing the stomach muscles back to normal. Breathing in comes naturally in this process. Keep contracting and relaxing the stomach muscles until the active exhalation and passive inhalation sound like bellows.

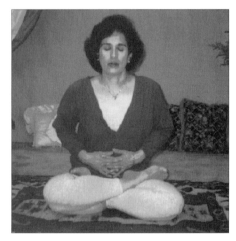

One round consists of 20 out and in breaths. (Depending on your ability and condition, practice for as little as a few breaths to as many as you can comfortably handle.) In the beginning, you may rest your palms on the abdomen in order to monitor the movements. After each round, lower your head and rest for about 10 seconds before starting the next round. Practice 3-5 rounds.

Benefits

Purifies the lungs. Quickly alleviates physical tiredness and mental fatigue. Boosts energy level. Activates the digestive system and tones the abdomen. Helps prevent and alleviate abdominal ailments, such as acidity, constipation, menstrual cramps, fibroid tumors, and toxic growths in the colon. Stimulates and uplifts the energy from the abdominal area to the heart center.

PANTING BREATH[6] (Bhastrika)

A quick and easy way to strengthen the lungs.

Practice

Sit comfortably with your back straight. Breathe in deeply. Breathe out and in rhythmically, compressing and expanding your chest evenly. One round is 20 out and in breaths. (Depending on your ability and condition, practice for as little as a few breaths to as many as you can.) After each round, lower your head and rest for about 10 seconds before starting the next round. Practice 3-5 rounds.

Benefits

Purifies, strengthens, and relaxes the lungs. Provides great benefits to runners, dancers, and other physically active individuals. Improves stamina.

---

[6] After a strenuous run, runners tend to open their mouth as they catch their breath. This technique is very similar to the way runners breathe, except that the mouth is closed. Regular practice of panting breath enables runners to recover their breath quickly.

LION BREATH (Simha)

A treat for the lungs, throat, and face!

Practice

Sit comfortably with your back straight. Breathe in and open your mouth wide. While looking upward, extend your tongue out as far as possible. Breathe out and in, as in panting breath, but with a slight roaring sound of a lion. Practice for 10-15 seconds. This is one round. Repeat 2-3 times.

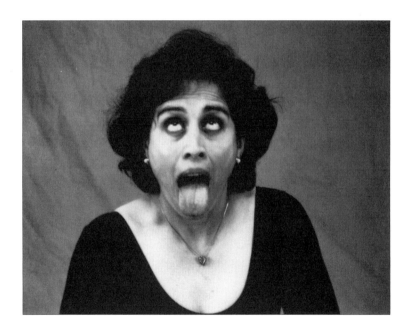

Benefits

Exercises and purifies the lungs. Alleviates and prevents sore throat and lung ailments. Massages the vocal chords. Stretches and firms the facial muscles, and relaxes the eyes. Reduces facial wrinkles.

COOLING BREATH (Sheetali)

A great aid to stop smoking and other addictive habits.

Practice

Sit comfortably with your back straight. Open your mouth slightly and curl your tongue up on both sides to form a hollow tube. Breathe in slowly through the tube. Close your mouth and swallow your breath. Hold the breath for a few seconds or for a comfortable duration. Breathe out slowly through your nose. This is one round. Practice 3-5 rounds.

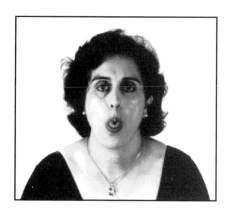

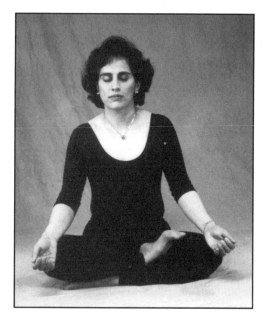

Benefits

Cools the whole system. Revitalizes every cell in the body.   Purifies the blood. Removes heat from the body, providing relief for hot flashes. Provides an excellent treatment for addictive habits, helping to reverse drug, alcohol, smoking, caffeine, and other undesirable addictions.

ENERGY RENEWING BREATHING[7] (Ujjayi)

A quick way to relax the endocrine system.

Practice

Sit comfortably with your back straight. Close your eyes. Rest the tip of your tongue on the upper palate. Close your lips. Breathe in and out slowly and deeply through your nose. Practice for about 2 minutes. In the beginning, you may find it difficult to hold the tip of your tongue in place. If this occurs, take short breaks and relax your tongue before repeating this technique. With practice, you can slide your tongue further towards the throat to experience immense benefits.

Benefits

Improves concentration; unfolds the hidden wisdom. Stimulates various pressure points and glands in the neck, which have extensive control over the activities of the body. Activates salivary glands. Relieves the feeling of thirst.

---

[7] This technique can be combined with 'healing by visualization' to provide instant relief for digestive and nervous disorders. For example, if you experience acidity or chest pain, practice energy renewing breathing while focussing on the pain-ridden area. Slightly emphasize the exhalation while visualizing the tension and pain leaving your body along with the breath. For detailed information on the 'healing by visualization' technique, refer to Chapter 3 on meditation.

BEE SOUNDING BREATH (Brahmari)

A soothing vibration for the brain.

Practice

Sit comfortably with your back straight. Maintain a slight gap between your upper and lower jaws as shown. Bringing your lips together, breathe in through your nose and hold your breath. (You may plug your ears with your index finger to intensify the vibration in your head.) While keeping your lips closed, gently make a humming or 'mmmmm' sound while allowing the air to flow out naturally through your nose. This is one round. Repeat 3-5 times. Rest for about 10-15 seconds.

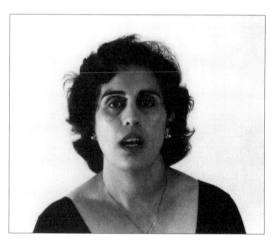 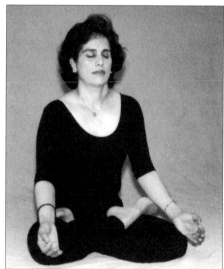

Benefits

Vibrates and revitalizes the brain cells, providing a soothing effect on the mind. Vibrates the throat, helping to alleviate and prevent colds, coughs, and sore throats. Massages the vocal chords, helping to improve the voice. Reduces blood pressure, and transforms anxiety into relaxation.

OM CHANTING

Brings immediate peace!

Practice

Sit comfortably with your back straight. Breathe in deeply through your nose. Pause for a moment. Start the om chanting, with the 'oooooo' sound, while allowing air to flow out naturally through your nose and mouth. With your mouth closed, finish the round with the 'mmmmm' sound, still breathing out through the nose. This comprises one round. Practice 5 to 6 rounds or as many as you wish.

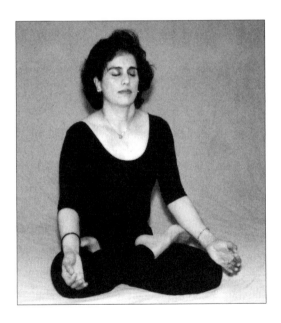

Benefits

Encourages deep breathing. Vibrates and relaxes the entire system. Promotes peace and inner joy. Develops a sense of unity and respect.

CORPSE RELAXATION (Shavasana)

The easiest and most comfortable pose for total relaxation!

This relaxation technique can be practiced by anyone, regardless of age or physical condition. It can also be practiced as an individual relaxation technique.

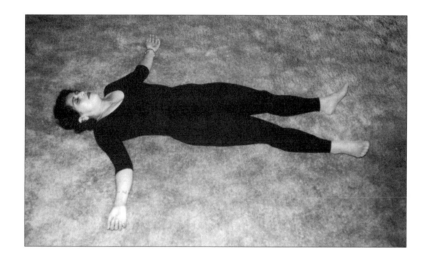

One of the most important benefits of this practice is that it can be practiced independent of any of the other yoga or pranayama techniques. For example, when you feel stressed or tired, just lie down and practice corpse relaxation. You may choose any one of the following practices to suit your needs.

Practice A (Full Body Awareness)

Lie down comfortably. Rest your arms slightly away from your body with your palms facing up and fingers loose. Keep your legs slightly apart and your feet relaxed, flopping to the side. Close your eyes. Focus your awareness on your natural breath. As you relax, slightly deepen your breathing by prolonging your exhalation while pulling your stomach muscles in. As you breathe in, let your pulled in stomach come up naturally and breathe upward while expanding your chest sideways. Breathe out from your chest to your stomach while pulling your stomach in as slowly as possible. Continue breathing slowly and deeply. Gradually allow your breath to return to natural breathing.

As you breathe naturally, shift your awareness to your face. Allow your forehead, eyes (open wide and then close), nose, cheeks, mouth (open wide and then close), and chin to relax. Shift your awareness from your face to your neck. Gently, roll your head to the right and then to the left several times, pausing for a few moments on each side. Allow your awareness to flow from your neck to your upper back and down to your shoulders, elbows, forearms, palms, and fingers. Continue breathing naturally for about 15 seconds. Next, shift your awareness to the expansion and compression of your chest and abdominal area and breathe slightly deeper for several breaths. Return to your natural breathing and focus on relaxing your spine, lower back, hips, thighs, knees, calves, ankles, heels, feet, and toes.

Focus your awareness on your entire body and just allow yourself to relax for a few moments. As you breathe in, feel the relaxation all over your body, in each and every cell. As you breathe out, release any stress, uneasiness, or tension remaining in your body. Relax your mind by being present in these relaxing moments. Let your mind flow along with your breath and relax deeply for as long as you want.

Practice B (Relaxation for a Specific Area)

Lie down and relax as in Practice A. When your body is relaxed, focus your awareness on any part of your body that is tense. Breathe naturally as you concentrate on that specific area. As you breathe out, feel the tension or uneasiness leave your body with your breath. As you breathe in, feel the energy flow to that part of your body. Keep practicing until you feel totally relaxed.

Practice C (Tension Release)

Lie down as in Practice A. Breathe in deeply. Hold your breath and tense the whole body by stretching your legs, feet, and arms while making tight fists. Slightly lift your arms as you tense them. Release the tension as you breathe out. Rest your arms. Repeat 3 to 4 times. Now allow your mind to enjoy this relaxation with slow steady breathing.

Benefits

Relaxes the entire body after strenuous exercise. Beneficial between yoga warm-ups, asanas, pranayama, and meditation. Releases physical, mental, and emotional tension. When practiced with focused awareness, this can be the foundation for creative self-healing. Refer to Chapter 3 on meditation for a detailed description of visualization and healing techniques.

ROUTINES

GENERAL ROUTINES

You may practice any one of the routines as shown or all the breathing techniques in the sequence in which they appear in this chapter.

ROUTINE 1

Simple breathing

Sniffing A and B

Rhythmic breathing

Bee sounding breath

Energy renewing breathing

Alternate nostril breathing

Corpse relaxation

ROUTINE 3

Simple breathing

Complete breathing

Bellows breath

Alternate nostril breathing

Energy renewing breathing

Om chanting

ROUTINE 2

Simple breathing

Complete breathing

Bellows breath

Panting breath

Lion breath

Double breath

Corpse relaxation

ROUTINES FOR SPECIFIC AILMENTS

High blood pressure

(**Note:** Do not practice breath retention.)

Simple breathing

Complete breathing

Alternate nostril breathing (A)

Bee sounding breath

Om chanting

Corpse relaxation for 15-20 minutes (A and B)

Low blood pressure

(**Note:** You may practice breath retention.)

Simple breathing

Complete breathing

Alternate nostril breathing (A, B, C or D)

Rhythmic breathing

Bee sounding breath

Om chanting

Corpse relaxation for 10-15 minutes (A or C)

Allergy or lung ailments

Simple breathing

Complete breathing

Alternate nostril breathing (include chin lock and breath retention)

Bellows breath

Lion breath

Om chanting

Corpse relaxation for 10-15 minutes (A or B)

Headaches

Simple breathing

Complete breathing

Alternate nostril breathing (include chin lock and breath retention)

Rhythmic breathing

Bee sounding breath

Corpse relaxation for 10-15 minutes (A, B, and C)

Abdominal ailments

Simple breathing

Complete breathing (emphasize the exhalations)

Bellows breath

Energy renewing breathing

Corpse relaxation for 15-20 minutes (A and B)

Hot flashes

Complete breathing (emphasize the exhalations)

Alternate nostril breathing

Cooling breath

Insomnia

Simple breathing

Rhythmic breathing

Complete breathing

Alternate nostril breathing

Corpse relaxation for 15-20 minutes (A and C)

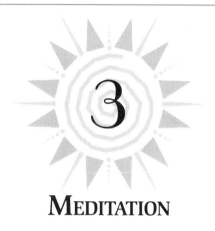

MEDITATION

"When we are at peace with ourselves, everything looks and feels beautiful."

Meditation is the practice of mindfulness--living with awareness. When we live with awareness, we are able to feel, reflect, and experience everything wholeheartedly. We pay closer attention to everything we do, down to the smallest detail. In this way, meditation becomes a continuous flow of awareness toward the subject of our observation.

Because the practice of meditation exists in many religions and has many different names, people have many misconceptions about what meditation really is, what it is not, and the manner in which it is practiced. The Hindus call mediation Dhyana; the Buddhists call it Ghana (Shene); the Japanese call it Zazen; the Christians call it contemplative prayer, and the Native Americans call it 'listening.' Whatever religion a particular technique of meditation originates from, the ultimate goal of all forms of meditation is to experience a quiet and peaceful state of mind in order to achieve a higher state of consciousness. Contrary to many common practices, the objective of meditation is NOT to achieve a blank space or a specific thought by blocking, suppressing, and neglecting our concerns. It is not the blank space we see when we close our eyes. Many people wish to set aside their stress and try to relax by merely focusing on an object or by visualizing that they are at a favorite vacation spot. In this process, the suppressed thoughts and feelings eventually resurface and accumulate in different parts of the body, causing further stress and illness. The first prerequisite for successful meditation is to balance the emotional and mental states. When the mind is balanced, deeper meditation comes naturally without struggle. We experience feelings of happiness, fulfillment, contentment, and inner peace when we close our eyes and integrate our body, mind, and breath. This state of being is something so beautiful and profound (transcendental) that it cannot be easily explained; it must be experienced. The method of meditation described in this chapter focuses on relaxing and quieting the mind by preparing the body through yogic exercise, and uniting the mind, body, and breath through conscious breathing. This method can be described as "quiet mind" training.

The mind is one of the most powerful things we possess. The mind interprets our experiences, allowing us to feel happy or sad, excited or depressed, challenged or overwhelmed, organized or scattered, and many other feelings. The mind also records all of our experiences from childhood to the present day whether the experience is positive or negative. You experience this power of the mind when a particular smell, color, sound, or event instantly triggers a memory from the past. For example, a particular aroma may take you back in time to feel nostalgic about your grandmother's cooking, a specific moment in your childhood, or a certain past experience with a friend or relative who now lives far away. The mind is so incredibly powerful that in just a few moments one can ponder many thoughts pertaining to the past, present, and future.

Good memories bring happiness, while memories of disappointments, uncertainties, or failures bring us unhappiness and upset our emotions. In order to avoid the past, some people suppress memories and feelings of unhappiness throughout their entire lives. These suppressed memories often emerge as tension, exhaustion, anger, guilt, or depression. People may also act out their suppressed feelings and memories in inappropriate ways or situations with other people. Such actions further exhaust the mind and affect the emotions which can lead to various types of illnesses. In extreme cases, this mental and emotional exhaustion may even cause people to harm others.

Meditation encourages us to take time out from our busy lives to observe and contemplate our experiences, so we can relax the mind and stabilize our emotions. When the mind is at peace and our emotions are balanced, we begin to become aware of the supreme power that is inherent in each one of us. This power guides us to understand ourselves and improve our self-esteem as well as understand and respect others.

Meditation improves concentration and naturally allows the memory of experiences to spring forth for review. As the experiences come forth, it is a time to tune into ourself and connect with our inner wisdom. Answers to questions appear automatically, priorities magically find their place, and challenges get resolved quietly and peacefully.

Meditation calms the restless, untrained, confused, and wandering mind. It helps us gain control over the expression of our emotions, so we can handle many situations that may have overwhelmed us in the past. Meditation also helps us develop an open mind and positive attitude so that we can cope with the stress in our lives.

Furthermore, meditation improves memory, replenishes energy levels, and boosts will power. It helps us develop a capacity for love, compassion, forgiveness, and serenity. These qualities help us release our egos and develop humility, along with a helping nature. Eventually, the cleansing and purification of the mind and body leads to higher consciousness and enlightened spirituality.

Meditation also helps balance our mental and physical energies. This, in turn, helps to improve our well-being while preventing or healing various ailments.

Although the specific purpose for which one practices meditation may vary from person to person, the results naturally lead to a variety of benefits.

STRESS MANAGEMENT

A common question from my students is "How can I get rid of my stress, insomnia, neck or back pain? Even though I have been practicing meditation and know how to achieve emptiness by not thinking about anything during meditation, I am still unable to relax and concentrate. I seem to always feel anxious, uneasy, and distracted. Is there any other method you can teach me that will help?" My answer is yes—meditate by focusing on your breath. Free your mind by allowing your thoughts to come forth by not suppressing them.

Swami Satyananda Saraswati placed great emphasis on freeing the mind through the process of meditation. "Purifying the mind is freeing the unwanted thoughts. It is not done by suppressing the various thoughts like anger, fear, disappointments, conflicts, worries, hatred, or any other. We have to deal with these feelings to eliminate them from our system. Suppressing our thoughts is harmful to our system and causes nervousness, guilt, rejection, and worthlessness in our daily lives. It is something like having diarrhea or a bad stomach and trying to control it. Of course, going to the toilet frequently can be very tiring. But ultimately, it will relax the whole stomach. We may take strong medicines to stop the purging, but then boils may erupt or other toxic side effects may arise. It is the same with the mind. Suppressing thoughts is like trying to hide our sorrow and uneasiness inside." Suppressed emotions either manifest as illness or lead to inappropriate thoughts or actions, thereby making matters worse.

Commonly, thoughts of job, family, and friends surface in meditation. For example, mothers may have thoughts about their children or students may be concerned about their assignments. Do not suppress any thoughts. Rather, take time to understand the nature of these thoughts and attune to what your inner wisdom tells you, as it is a powerful guiding force. Meditation has helped me to be a gentle, loving, and understanding parent as well as to act with patience in stressful situations.

PHYSICAL HEALTH

Generally, people who practice yoga and meditation regularly are able to completely balance their emotions and maintain their health. This does not mean that yoga and meditation practitioners do not get sick. When they do get sick, they usually have the ability to recover quickly as they have an abundance of prana in their systems. One's state of health depends on the individual and how well he or she practices these techniques.

Michele Moreland, a law student, explains, "I try to begin my day by practicing yoga and meditation. The days I do not practice I am noticeably less energetic, less relaxed, and more irritable. Through the postures, pranayama, and meditation, I can check in with my body and my emotions, deal with problems and tension, or just feel good about having gotten up early to do yoga. The amazing thing about it - aside from feeling happier and less stressful - is that I can actually prevent sickness. In the past, I typically had three or four sinus infections a year, a migraine headache every couple of months, and frequent colds. I haven't had one sinus infection all year since I began practicing and have had only one migraine, and a couple of colds. Also, my body is more toned—without even entering a gym!"

Mohanlal Sharma, a retired vice principal, says, "For the last two years I have been attending yoga classes conducted by Vasanthi Bhat. In the morning, I regularly practice yogic exercises for one hour and meditation for 15 minutes besides brisk morning walks. I regulated my diet by avoiding fatty foods and oily substances and concentrating on low-fat milk, fruit juices, and laxative vegetables. The results are evident: digestion has improved, arthritis pain has subsided, blood pressure is under control, body weight has decreased by ten pounds, and cholesterol count has declined from 229 to 180 mg/dl. I am grateful to Vasanthi, who has given me an opportunity to experience healthy living at this young age of 75."

WEIGHT CONTROL

Some of my students use yoga and meditation for the purpose of weight loss. When I was overweight, the first thought that used to come to my mind when I was meditating was "How am I going to lose weight?" I did not neglect this thought but focused on it, seeking advice from within. I got all the positive answers I needed to help me. Answers like "Pay attention to what you eat," "Be more active," "Do deep breathing, stretching, and brisk walking," and "Never give up." All these answers came to me as I was breathing deeply in my meditation. The practice of deep breathing is one of the most important techniques for weight loss. The higher the level of prana in our systems, the easier it is to tap into our inner wisdom to boost our energy levels and self-esteem.

Smitha Uttarwar, a young student of mine, wanted to lose weight. She recalls, "I have been studying yoga with Vasanthi for three years now. I recall when I first came to Vasanthi after doing yoga for a month. I asked her, 'Vasanthi, can you help me? I want to lose weight. Can I do it?' She said, 'Of course.' She also gave me a few hints about diet along with practice techniques. She suggested cutting down on oil, adding more vegetables and fruits to my diet. 'If you feel like eating a cake or any favorite food, go ahead and enjoy it with a full mind. But try to not go to extremes. Adopt in moderation any style that you can continue happily.' I did just that, along with 45 minutes of yoga postures, breathing, and meditation every day. Believe it or not, I lost 40 pounds in five to six months. I am happy, energetic and full of strength now. Because of yoga, I have been able to maintain my weight. When I visited India after having lost weight, my father, who is a doctor, was both surprised and happy, but was also rather concerned to find me so skinny. He insisted on putting me through a full examination. First, I had a blood test and then a physical. Everything came out perfectly. He said, 'Smitha, you lost so much weight in such a short time and yet stayed healthy. It must be the food you ate, as well as your yoga, breathing, and meditation practice'."

CONCENTRATION

Alina Shah, a sixth-grade student, attends my classes to alleviate her allergies and improve her concentration.

Ashwini Ranjan, a 12 year-old, also practices yoga to enhance her concentration. "My interest in yoga began when my friend Alina Shah mentioned to me that yoga lessons had been very beneficial to her. Although I have started learning yoga from Vasanthi Bhat only recently, the advantages are already apparent to me. Yoga meditation has made me relax and has improved my memory and concentration skills. I look forward to my yoga lessons every week and intend to keep yoga as a part of my everyday routine in the future."

ENERGIZING

Many of my students express great happiness at being more energetic after practicing yoga and meditation. Many senior students over 70 years of age tell me that they feel so energetic as if they were in their early thirties!

LIVING IN THE PRESENT

Students commonly ask, "How can I live in the present if my mind is constantly wandering?" The answer is to meditate on those wandering thoughts. Focus your awareness on such thoughts and eventually the nature of the thoughts will be clear. The mind generally wanders when we accumulate too many doubts or uncertainties about our past experiences or our immediate duties to be performed. We waste an enormous amount of energy and time by just worrying about past and future events. This does not mean that we should not think of them, because we do have to plan our future and think of the past in order to do better. Learning from our past experiences and planning the future can be part of our meditation, helping us to make the best out of the present moment. For example, when practicing yoga, some common thoughts that distract the mind may be, "What am I going to cook," "What am I going to buy tomorrow," or "What does my boss want?" Sometimes past memories come up. By the end of our yoga practice, we may have been unable to enjoy the stretching moments because we were mentally preoccupied. During mealtimes, the mind may wander, thinking of the next day's exercise practice or the activities planned for the day. In this process, even though we satisfy our appetite, we are unable to relish the taste of the food we have consumed. On the whole, the ability to live in the present is missing along with our ability to benefit from these activities. If you breathe consciously when distracting thoughts appear, you will be able to prioritize your flow of thoughts. If you feel they are really important, you may analyze these disturbing thoughts while meditating on them (refer to vipasana meditation). You will find solutions to these thoughts by living in the present. This will make you happy as it allows you to continue with your present activity with total awareness.

Unless we overcome our mental distractions, there will be no end to the wandering of the mind. Constantly living either in the past or in the future prevents us from being aware of our present, and we end up missing out on many things in our present life. The more time we take to understand and prioritize the nature of our thoughts, the easier it is for the mind to be in the present moment in order to absorb, enjoy, learn, correct, and appreciate.

Another example of people missing the present moments is when they concentrate on reading while exercising in the gym. They can obtain greater benefits from the workout if they meditate by breathing consciously, while focusing on the current activity for their specific needs. Their inability to focus leads to muscular and mental tension as the present body condition is neglected. As a result, many people injure their back, knees, or other parts while exercising. Very often, this is not due to the exercise itself, but due to the lack of attention to the condition of the body during the activity. When one's mind is not completely focussed on the current activity, one tends to ignore, overwork, and injure the muscles.

SPIRITUALITY

Different people have different interpretations of God and therefore, follow different paths to attain spirituality. Some people visualize pictures of deities; others practice chanting. Some like Mother Theresa helped the poor or needy. Others develop their spirituality by saying a quick prayer before performing an activity. No matter how one practices, unless one is able to find one's inner power by balancing the emotions, it will be difficult to achieve inner peace. Inner peace or power is the same in everyone, whether young or old, rich or poor.

We are all born with supreme power within us, and we die when it leaves the body. Our breath or prana is the link to this spiritual power. It is a universal energy that is always available. If we meditate on our spiritual power or prana, we can experience and create many good things. This spiritual meditation leads to inner peace and improved self-esteem, and expands our respect and love for all. **Respecting and loving everyone regardless of age, race, religion, and status is spirituality.**

Swami Sivananda said, "Every person has good and bad qualities. In order to purify the bad thoughts or actions, one needs to meditate on them. Spiritual meditation is very powerful because you have a direct connection to God, the power or energy within you or your inner self." We can act, cheat, or lie, but we cannot deny our inner consciousness. It keeps disturbing our mental peace. So attaining the spiritual level means purifying our inner consciousness, which directly influences our actions. It is not how many hours we sit or stand near an idol of God and pray. It is how often we take time to purify ourselves. Swami Sivananda stressed the importance of mentally chanting a mantra whenever possible in order to purify the mind and guide our actions.

There are many different techniques for practicing meditation, some of which are described in this chapter. You may adapt any one or more of these techniques to suit your convenience, place, and available time. You can practice these methods separately or as part of the hatha yoga sequence of asana, pranayama, and meditation. Choose the practice that best meets your needs. Advanced practitioners can combine meditation with their asanas and pranayama to experience intense benefits and emotional stability.

Meditation Practice	Benefits
Vipasana meditation	Purifies and balances the emotions.
Meditation in the postures	Balances physical, mental, and emotional energy. Stimulates the chakras.
Meditation during pranayama	Purifies the emotions and improves concentration.
Healing by visualization or Pranic healing meditation	Helps prevent and heal ailments.
Yoga nidra meditation	Develops connection with inner power.
Meditation towards success	Helps achieve goals.
Karma yoga	Brings spirituality to our daily duties.
Everyday meditation	Helps bring positive changes in our life-style.

THINGS TO KNOW BEFORE PRACTICING MEDITATION

- Meditation can be practiced from a few seconds to as long as you like. It is a learning process that takes time, patience, experience, and understanding yourself and others. Everyday is a learning process because everyday you encounter different people, different situations, and new challenges. What works one day may not be the solution another day. But remember, each time you practice meditation with an open mind, regardless of the place or length of your practice, you will learn about life and gain new levels of experience.

- It is best to sit straight with the base of your spine resting firmly on the floor. Sitting comfortably with a straight spine has a direct effect on your concentration and helps quiet the mind. It is not necessary to sit in the full or half lotus positions in order to meditate. In fact, some meditation does not even require sitting. Zen meditators do a very slow walking meditation called "kinnon." Chi Kung meditators sometimes do a standing meditation while facing the sun. Tibetan Buddhists practice a form of meditation while standing on the tips of their toes with arms in the air over their heads. Yoga meditators meditate in their favorite posture or pose, one of which is the lotus or half lotus sitting position. At its very finest and most advanced state, meditation can be practiced all the time, while taking a walk, eating a meal, or doing any activity. My comfortable meditative positions are the lotus, shoulder stand, plough, and pose of the moon as well as their variations. Many of my students like to meditate in their favorite poses such as pose of the moon, turtle, plough, and others. However, you may adopt any comfortable position to practice meditation.

- You may sit in simple cross-legged (sukhasana), half-lotus (siddhasana), full lotus (padmasana), or sitting on the heels (vajrasana). You could be sitting in a chair or a comfortable yoga pose. Refer to Chapter 2 for a description of different sitting positions. Another position that is preferred is to stretch one leg in front of you, slightly bent at the knee, and position the opposite foot near the thigh. You may use a cushion to sit on or lean against the wall. If your condition does not allow you to assume any of the above positions, feel free to sit or lie down anywhere you wish. It is very important to find a position you can sit in comfortably, so that you can develop the discipline and concentration to meditate.

- Remember, the mind and body work together. For example, think of your first reaction when you feel uneasiness in any part of your body. You immediately begin to think about the uneasiness instead of maintaining the meditative state. So the moment the body is not comfortable, it affects your concentration. Therefore, in order to bring your mind back to a meditative state, it is important to relax the body. When the body is relaxed, so is the mind. With a relaxed body, you will naturally fall into a meditative state.

- In the beginning of your practice, you may get distracted by various thoughts. You may think of your health, job, family, friends, or have other distracting thoughts. You might feel uneasiness in your body. Just remember, this is the beginning of your meditation and the beginning of understanding yourself. When your mind wanders, gently bring it back to the present. If you are uncomfortable, make yourself comfortable. If you are restless, practice simple breathing. However, if the distracting thoughts keep recurring, do not try to suppress or ignore them. This will cause inner stress and anxiety. Entertain these thoughts and begin to study them by analyzing the cause of the thoughts and allow your inner wisdom to respond appropriately.

- Remember to check your breath while practicing meditation. Often you may focus on an object or thought and forget your breath. Proper breathing is the key to successful meditation.

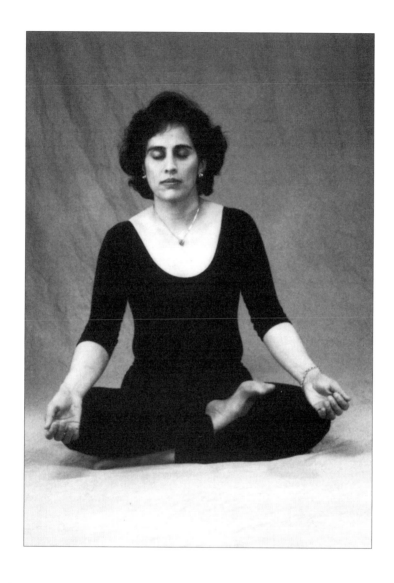

MEDITATION PRACTICE

VIPASANA MEDITATION (Antar Mouna or Inner Silence)

Vipasana meditation is practiced while keeping awareness towards your natural breath. During vipasana meditation, you quietly observe, express, open up, analyze, and find solutions to your concerns. As the concerns are resolved and unpleasant thoughts are eliminated, the mind becomes calm and experiences inner peace.

Practice

Sit comfortably with your eyes closed. Shift your awareness towards your natural breathing. Do not change your breathing pattern. Simply experience your breath flowing through your nostrils and its effects on your system. Try to be conscious of the present moment. If your mind starts wandering, do not feel that you are meditating incorrectly because it is normal for the mind to wander. Do not block or suppress any thoughts; at the same time do not invite them.

You may be surprised by how many diverse thoughts come and go. Thoughts are just stored memories or impressions. Just continue the meditation with an open mind and observe the thoughts closely as they arise from the subconscious mind. Good and bad thoughts may arise. Bad impressions must be eliminated from your mind to purify your system. Analyze a particular thought if it disturbs you emotionally. Otherwise, just let it pass. Meditating on a particular thought might help you find solutions. Do not be disappointed if one particular thought or issue takes longer to solve than others. Try to meditate everyday for at least 10-15 minutes to find positive answers to your concerns. Once you find positive answers, these thoughts will not disturb you anymore.

We often feel sad while remembering past events or worrying about our future. This causes anxiety and depression, and upsets our emotions. Swami Sivananda emphasized the need to often take a few moments to balance our emotions. We cannot change the past. But it is in our capacity to change our future or destiny. To change the future, we have to act right now by changing our attitude. Often, we are depressed about the things we did not do right, and we continue to worry about them.

Utilize your past experiences to change your present attitude by meditating on your mistakes to learn something beneficial from them. Often, they can reveal important things to avoid in the future or important considerations. To your surprise, as answers and ideas come forth, a particular disturbing thought will soon disappear. Even if it comes back, it will have a diminished effect, and over time such thoughts will naturally disappear from your system. This does not mean that you will not recall the thought some day; however, if you do recall the thought, it will not have any effect on your emotions.

The nature of your thoughts depends on your current and past situations. Some thoughts can be complicated, distressed, angry, hateful, and pessimistic. Remember, a particular thought or problem might take a few days, a few months, or even years for your inner wisdom to find an appropriate answer. Also, understand that as long as you have ongoing interaction with different people, you will always have new issues to take care of.

Sometimes, we make mistakes or offend others without realizing it. We waste an enormous amount of energy by holding on to our 'egos'. Vipasana meditation is a wonderful technique to loosen up the 'ego'.

Meditate faithfully. Remember, you know yourself best! For example, the issue could be an unpleasant argument or miscommunication between spouses, parents, children, friends, or co-workers. It is natural that interactions sometimes lead to miscommunications. Unless you deal with situations squarely and express your opinions honestly, they will continue to cause tension, which in turn will disturb your emotions. This becomes an obstacle for inner purification and attaining a higher level of consciousness. Now the question is "Who is going to make the effort?" You are, of course!

When we fail to make an effort, we harbor thousands of unresolved issues in our system. Consequently, we develop hatred towards others. This can be a major obstacle in our efforts to achieve inner peace because disturbing thoughts can be a constant distraction. When we are purified, we experience such peace of mind that nothing disturbs us anymore. This purified mind enables us to deal with issues or problems promptly. This is when we are capable of experiencing the so called blank space **chidakash** where thoughts just come and go without affecting our emotions. This is a peaceful meditative state. In this state of mind, we start appreciating the simple pleasures in life, such as nature, colors, the place where we live, and other creations of God. We begin to understand and appreciate what we have in life, rather than thinking about what we do not have. We also learn to understand the difficulties of others as if they are our own. These are some of the aspects of the spiritual path towards self-realization.

Utilize these precious moments to chant or express thanks to God. The mind transcends to a state of selflessness, evoking love, compassion, forgiveness, and positive thinking. In this state, you regain an abundance of energy and wish to utilize it positively. You might wonder from where all this positive energy and happiness come. They were dormant within you all along!

MEDITATION IN THE POSTURES

This meditation technique is for those who prefer to meditate in the yoga poses.

Practice

You can either adopt your favorite asana or meditate as you practice your yoga routine. If you are physically tense or need to stretch tired muscles, you may meditate towards the stretching effects, visualize and concentrate on specific parts of your body to obtain healing effects, or take time to observe your emotions (vipasana meditation) as they reveal themselves.

Meditating in the asanas allows you to understand your physical limits, thereby avoiding unnecessary force. When you are very comfortable in the asanas, your breath flows freely. This naturally helps release accumulated physical (muscular), mental, and emotional tension. Remember, it is normal for the mind to get distracted if you are not comfortable in the pose. Focussing on the effects of the poses also helps control the wandering mind.

When your body and mind are relaxed, your breath begins to flow freely. This balances the energy in the ida and pingala nadis (sympathetic and para-sympathetic nerves). In this balanced state, you experience the awakening of the kundalini energy by energizing the sushumna channel (located in the central spine). The awakened kundalini rises from the mooladhara chakra (near the base of the spine) and unites in the sahasrara (center of higher consciousness) allowing you to experience bliss and tranquility. In this state, you move closer to your higher consciousness (soul) as your mind no longer wanders. You experience contentment, happiness, and bliss. In this state, you will naturally want to chant mantras or thank God. This further unfolds the hidden power, helping you to live positively. Therefore, relaxing the body while balancing the prana in the sympathetic and para-sympathetic nervous system (ida and pingala channels) is one of the most important steps in **hatha yoga** to achieve this balanced state of consciousness.

Chakra	Location	Quality
Sahasrara	Top of the Head	Higher Consciousness
Ajna	Between the Eyebrows	Concentration & Intuition
Vishuddhi	Thyroid Area	Purification
Anahata	Heart	Love & Compassion
Manipura	Abdominal Area	Digestion & Abdominal Activities
Swadhisthana	Base of the Spine	Reproductive System
Mooladhara	Between Rectum and Base of the Spine	Kundalini Energy

Generally, backward bending poses help tap and release energy from the mooladhara chakra (rectal region) to the swadhisthana chakra (base of the spine), manipura chakra (stomach), and upwards. If you constantly have back pain or abdominal ailments and stomach disorders, it is advisable to practice backward bending poses followed by forward bending poses and spinal twists to relax and release the energy upward. If you do not take care of this, it is an obstacle to good health because energy (prana) gets blocked in that area. When the energy does not flow above the stomach center, you tend to have negative thoughts and outlooks, which affect your health and well-being.

Forward bending and inverted poses followed by spinal twists help direct energy from the manipura (stomach) upward to the anahata (heart), vishuddhi (neck), and ajna (concentration) chakras. For heart ailments and emotional disturbances, practice forward bending and inverted poses followed by backward bending poses and spinal twists. This helps release and balance the energy in all the centers and further directs it to the ajna (concentration) and sahasrara (higher consciousness) chakras. This naturally helps improve concentration and develop love, compassion, and forgiveness (eliminating ego and hatred), leading to a more positive outlook.

Therefore, in order to stimulate the chakras, it is important to be fully conscious of your physical condition while meditating in the postures. The full impact of this transcendental state can be understood only when you experience it.

MEDITATION DURING PRANAYAMA

Structured counting and mantra chanting techniques are for those who prefer to meditate while practicing pranayama. These techniques can also be practiced prior to vipasana meditation to calm your restless or wandering mind.

The following counting or chanting (the mental repetition of any word) meditation will tremendously improve your concentration and will power.

Pranayama meditation increases your awareness towards your breath flow. This naturally helps you focus on your eyebrow center (ajna chakra). This will enable the practitioner to concentrate, as one of the characteristics of this center is concentration.

When practiced with complete breathing and bellows breath pranayama, this meditation helps release and uplift the kundalini energy from the stomach to the higher centers. However, the uplifting of energy can only occur when you are physically comfortable. Any discomfort in any part of the body prevents the energy from being released.

When practiced with alternate nostril breathing including the chin lock and rectal contraction, this meditation is the most powerful technique for balancing the flow of energy in the ida and pingala (sympathetic and parasympathetic nervous systems). This balanced flow of energy encourages the kundalini energy to flow freely through the chakras. For additional benefit, you may visualize the flow of energy to a particular chakra as you meditate with the breath flow. You can also focus on the chakras in ascending and descending order to experience the power of the kundalini energy and its effects on your mind.

Practice A (Simple Breath Counting)

Sit comfortably with your eyes closed. Focus towards your natural, effortless breathing. When your breath is steady, begin the meditation by mentally counting each breath. Remember that breathing in and breathing out is one breath. The next in and out breath cycle is counted as the second breath. Let the rhythm come naturally. Try to count 7-10 breaths. If you get lost, go back to the beginning of your count and start again. If you finish one round, you are doing great! Keep your goal of 7-10 breaths. When once you are comfortable with this technique, your natural breath begins to flow slowly and deeply. You can continue meditating on the deep breathing, increasing your goal to a comfortable number of 20, 30, or more breaths. Always meditate up to the point where your energy and emotions are balanced. It could be anywhere from a few breaths to as long as it takes.

Practice B (Double Exhalation)

Sit comfortably with your eyes closed. Focus towards your natural, effortless breathing. When your breath is steady, begin the counting meditation by selecting a comfortable breathing pattern. Allow your exhalation to be twice the duration of your inhalation, a ratio of 1:2. For example, breathe in for 2 seconds and breathe out for 4 seconds. Or breathe in for 3, 4, 5, or 6 seconds and breathe out for 6, 8, 10, or 12 seconds respectively. Once you are comfortable with this breathing technique, your exhalation naturally becomes twice the duration of your inhalation, even without counting. Practice this for about 10 breaths or as many as you wish.

Practice C (Structured Breath Counting)

Precautions: Please remind yourself to avoid straining in order to achieve perfect counting. Stop retaining the breath the moment you experience strain in your chest muscles. Pranayama is controlling the vital air in the body without strain or force.

Sitting comfortably with your eyes closed, focus towards your natural, effortless breathing. Use the tables below for practicing this breath counting meditation. Adopt a ratio that suits your comfort level (Chin lock and rectal contraction can be practiced in all the pranayama while retaining your breath). For example, breathe in for 2 seconds, hold for 2 seconds, and breathe out for 4 seconds (1:1:2 ratio). Or if you wish to practice greater retention, breathe in for 2 seconds, hold for 4 seconds, and breathe out for 4 seconds (1:2:2 ratio). Remember to pause slightly in between each step. For example, breathe in for 2 seconds, pause, hold for 2 seconds, pause, breathe out for 4 seconds, and pause.

Gradually progress to the 1:4:2 ratio.

1:1:2 Ratio

Breathe In	Hold	Breathe Out
2	2	4
3	3	6
4	4	8

1:2:2 Ratio

Breathe In	Hold	Breathe Out
2	4	4
3	6	6
4	8	8

1:4:2 Ratio

Breathe In	Hold	Breathe Out
2	8	4
3	12	6
4	16	8

Practice D (Alternate Nostril Breathing with Chin Lock and Rectal Contraction)

Initially, alternate nostril breathing can be practiced using the 1:1:2 ratio. After this is mastered, the 1:2:2 or 1:4:2 ratio may be adopted. Once you are comfortable with the breath retention, you may incorporate the chin lock and rectal contraction into your practice routine. Refer to Chapter 2 for detailed instructions.

Close your left nostril after breathing in. Hold your breath. While holding your breath, lower your head as you move your shoulders up. Slowly lower your chin to your chest. Practice rectal contraction and begin counting the retention. Release the contraction, lift your head, and breathe out through the right nostril. Now, breathe in through your right nostril, close, hold the breath, chin lock, rectal contraction, release, back to the upright position, and breathe out through your left nostril. This is one round. Repeat 3-5 rounds.

Practice E (Rhythmic Breath Counting)

Use the tables below to practice rhythmic breath counting meditation. Adopt a ratio that suits your comfort level. Remember to pause slightly between steps. Rectal contraction can also be practiced during breath retention.

1:1:1:1 Ratio

Breathe In	Hold	Breathe Out	Hold
2	2	2	2
3	3	3	3
4	4	4	4

1:2:1:2 Ratio

Breathe In	Hold	Breathe Out	Hold
2	4	2	4
3	6	3	6
4	8	4	8

Practice F (Chanting)

When your breath counting flows systematically, you can combine the counting with chanting. Mentally repeat your favorite word or mantra in place of numbers. For instance, words such as Om, peace, kind, moon, flower, a personal deity's name, or your favorite word[1] may be adopted. (Chanting improves concentration because you have to focus on the count as well as the mantra.) For example, om1, om2, om3, and so on.

With practice, you will be able to incorporate mantra chanting effortlessly anytime or anywhere, without following any breath-counting pattern. For example, mantra chanting can flow easily with your conscious breathing during asanas, your walk, or anytime. Mantra chanting is very powerful because it easily connects you to your higher self (soul). It also has an immediate soothing effect on your nervous system. It is like having a genuine friend within you all the time!

[1] Generally, if you keep practicing yoga, a suitable mantra will naturally unfold depending on your nature. In some places, Swamijis, gurus or learned individuals help people adopt mantras.

However, until you get your mantra, you may adopt a word that suits your needs. For example, if you experience nervousness, you may repeat a name (realized person, guru, or deity) or a word (relax, calm) that symbolizes or represents tranquility, calm, or peace. Another popular chant is So.... (as you breathe in) and Hum...m (as you breath out). Prolong the chant for the duration of your in and out breaths respectively, without maintaining a breath count.

Contrary to some opinions, there is no restriction in sharing your mantra with others.

HEALING BY VISUALIZATION (Pranic Healing Meditation)

Healing by visualization involves focusing your mind on the part of the body you wish to heal and directing the stimulating energy of your breath to that part of your body. This method of meditation can be practiced by people of all ages. It is also beneficial for those who are unable to do the postures because of physical limitations, injuries, internal problems, or physical weakness. Healing visualization can be practiced to either help treat specific ailments or help restore physical strength and health. This technique can be practiced in any position: sitting, lying down, practicing postures, and even while walking. However, lying down is the best position because your body is able to rest completely, allowing for improved concentration.

Practice

Adopt a comfortable position and close your eyes. Take a few moments to relax your body and mind as in corpse relaxation practice A or B in Chapter 2. When you have relaxed your mind and body, you are ready to direct prana to all or needed parts. First, bring your awareness to your right palm and fingers as you breathe. Feel the energy flow into your palm and each finger. Feel the relaxation in the muscles and heaviness in your hand. Now try the same technique for the left hand or any part of your body you wish to heal.

Focus your attention on the desired part of your body. For example, for arthritis, focus on your joints; for hypertension, focus on your heart; for asthma, focus on your lungs; for headaches, focus on your temples; for abdominal cramps, focus on your abdomen; for ulcers, focus on your stomach. Feel the energy flow to the chosen part and visualize the healing. As you breathe in, feel the flow of prana to the focused part of your body. As you breathe out, imagine the pain, tension, and strain leaving your body. The powerful stimulating energy of your breath releases the tension or stress from that part of the body and channels new revitalizing energy to that area. Also while breathing out, mentally repeat an affirmation like "I am getting rid of the uneasiness" and "I am getting better." Depending on the nature of the ailments, you have to think positively and appropriately. For example, if you wish to heal clogged arteries, visualize your heart and send energy to the coronary arteries, visualizing the arteries getting cleared of any blockages. If it is for an ulcer, visualize the ulcer getting smaller and leaving your system.

You can also utilize this method to lose weight by visualizing weight loss from a specific area of your body. Focus your attention on that part of your body while stretching or exercising for optimum benefit. Remember to practice this technique with faith and a positive attitude. This will enhance your workout and you will notice significant results.

Depending on the nature of your ailment, also remember to release the suppressed emotions as you are healing. For example, emotional tension can constrict the heart muscles. Abdominal ailments may be accompanied by mental tension.

Anjali Kiran, a graphic artist, shares, "I have been learning yoga from Vasanthi for the past 5 years. Yoga has not only helped me to be healthy physically but mentally as well. My most recent experience of yoga was during my last pregnancy. During the first trimester, I was diagnosed with a fibroid in my uterus. My doctor said that the presence of fibroid in many cases could lead to either a premature labor or a miscarriage. I was totally shaken up. The following Saturday, I met Vasanthi during our scheduled yoga class and shared the information with her. Vasanthi said, 'Do not worry about the problem. If you worry you will be under stress and things could get worse. But at the same time, you should not ignore the fibroid either. First be calm and do deep breathing exercises. Visualize your uterus and the fibroid. Using the picture of the ultrasound to locate the exact spot, send energy to the tumor and visualize that the fibroid is shrinking. Think beautiful thoughts of the baby growing within you.' She further recommended that I practice this for 10-15 minutes at a time, throughout the day – any place or any time. I practiced this throughout my pregnancy. My doctor was amazed with the results! I had a full term pregnancy and there are no traces of the fibroid now. Vasanthi's concern and appropriate guidance helped me a lot."

YOGA NIDRA MEDITATION (Yoga Sleep)

Yoga nidra meditation is considered a very advanced technique because it is hard to practice without falling asleep. With practice, yoga nidra can be experienced with total awareness, thereby maximizing its extremely powerful benefits.

Practice

Lie down with your arms resting slightly away from your body. With your palms facing up, relax your fingers. Rest your legs slightly apart and let your feet flop to the sides. Follow the corpse relaxation practice A described in Chapter 2. As you are practicing, take a few moments to respect and appreciate your body. Feel the revitalization in each and every cell of your body. Allow your mind to be with your present practice by focusing your awareness on your natural breath. As in the healing by visualization meditation, direct the prana to any tense muscles to relax further. Remember, more prana naturally flows to the area you are focusing on.

If your concentration is keenly focused and you are deeply connected to your subconscious mind, this is a time to listen to your inner voice (inner wisdom) and allow it to guide you. So, meditate on your wishes and how you may fulfil them. The subconscious mind is very receptive to your true wishes and will obediently help you carry them out. Listen attentively to the genuine answers from within and follow them accordingly to accomplish your goals. This has the same effect as hypnosis, except that it is self-directed by communicating with your subconscious mind. Depending on the nature of your wishes, it might take a few days, months, or even years to fulfil. Never give up!

MEDITATION TOWARDS SUCCESS

The first and most important step towards success is feeling that you can succeed. Success is not limited to grand accomplishments, but can involve activities like working around the house, bringing up children, respecting parents and friends, or performing an athletic activity. Try to live in the present moment and develop determination. Be persistent and do not give up until you find the answers or the results you desire.

Practice

Meditate on your success by thinking of all that you would like to accomplish, imagining that you have already accomplished your goals. Just imagining success feels good. Now, understand how hard you need to work in order to achieve this success. This is the most difficult and painful aspect because most of the time it is easier to give up the idea of success than it is to embrace the need for hard work. Instead of giving up on your success when faced with hard work, start by finding yourself a role model. This could be someone or several people who are successful in their work and who motivate you just by thinking about them. Get to know their life-styles and find out how much they have had to sacrifice towards their goals. When you get discouraged and do not want to put out any more effort, contemplate how each step, no matter how small, is leading toward your goal. Meditate while breathing consciously and ask yourself if this is the outcome you really want.

I often motivate myself by thinking of teenage gymnasts and figure skaters. These girls and boys have to be very self-motivated to practice for many hours. This is a great inspiration to me! When you do motivate yourself to work hard, make sure to acknowledge it by writing it down on a calendar or in your diary. Reward yourself for your efforts to motivate yourself further.

However, everyone makes mistakes and experiences failure. Persist in continuing towards your goals, although you have encountered failures and made mistakes. According to Saint Purandaradasa, "Whatever happens in life, it is for something good." It is also said that failures are stepping stones to success. With this attitude in mind, you can always learn something positive from your failures and mistakes. Use your failures and mistakes as keys to open other ideas and possibilities. When you are able to live in the present moment, good and positive guidance can come to you even in the worst situations. Worrying about the past is only going to de-motivate you, cause depression, and bring sorrow. Try to develop the courage to keep focused on your goals. All of your dreams can come true if you have the courage to pursue them. Remember to have faith in yourself.

Constantly remind yourself that you are unique in many ways. Find your unique nature and work hard until you achieve the results you desire. Resist comparing yourself to anyone. Just accept who you are and always respect your inner self, your views, and what your inner voice or wisdom tells you. Try not to change your personality to please others. This acceptance is a sign of self respect. Work hard to achieve your goals. Swami Sivananda said to my Guru Satyananda Saraswati when he joined the ashram, "Work hard to purify. And the light will unfold within you."

Therefore, in order to be successful, try to do your best while understanding the value and significance of your work. When you have done your best, simply reward yourself for your efforts. The reward could be just thinking good about yourself, buying affordable things, or even enjoying your favorite food. Remember to always express thanks and appreciation to God!

KARMA YOGA

Performing our duties faithfully without being attached to the outcome is karma yoga.

There are certain things in life that are fun to do. You do them joyfully and wholeheartedly. You have no trouble concentrating on them and many times do them with great creativity. There are also situations in life that are wonderful and rewarding to go through and you gladly embrace them.

However, the opposite is also true. When the "not so good" jobs and situations have to be dealt with, you may put them off or rebel and allow them to cause great stress in your life. You waste an enormous amount of energy building resistance to doing even the simplest bit of work when it is not of interest to you. Lack of enthusiasm in performing your duties leads to anger, depression, sleeplessness, and irritability. You may complain and whine, act depressed, and waste time procrastinating. This is when **Karma yoga** can play an important role in your life. If you change your attitude by giving importance to your work (good and not so good) as your enlightened or higher duty and meditate on the positive effects that your duties can lead to, everything changes. You no longer need to resist your duties, put them off, or cause stress and anger to yourself. Instead, you happily do it all and feel grateful to accept your roles. Performing your duties faithfully without expecting anything in return helps you restore the misused energy in your life and experience immense joy. You can then do any type or amount of work without getting tired because you will be able to utilize your energy positively and mindfully. In addition, your breathing is very relaxed and controlled while working. A steady breath further helps relax your mind, mend your attitude, and free you from unnecessary thoughts and resistance.

EVERYDAY MEDITATION

Now that you know basic meditation, practice your favorite techniques everyday from a few minutes to as long as you wish. In addition, try to utilize these meditation techniques throughout the day to revitalize yourself and live in the present moment. In other words, practice conscious breathing as much as possible to live with increased awareness. For example, practice conscious breathing while waking up, taking a shower, eating meals, or driving to work. I call it a 'handy' practice.

The following seven techniques are helpful ways for you to adopt meditation in your daily life. You will be surprised to experience and learn many different things each day. You will also notice positive changes in your life-style with reduced stress. When you master these meditation techniques, it will be very easy for you to incorporate meditation in your daily life. Basically, meditation becomes a part of your life.

Upon Waking Up

When you wake up in the morning and are still in bed, close your eyes and try to practice slow, controlled breathing while praying or chanting your mantra for a few minutes. Do not let stressful thoughts take over these precious moments. Give yourself positive encouragement and affirmation. Adopt a 'karma yoga' attitude and thank God for His guidance.

Sun Bathing

Sunrise or sunset are the best times to spend a few moments with nature while practicing your favorite yoga techniques, such as bellows breath, alternate nostril breathing, double angle pose, and toe stretching. It takes only a few minutes to absorb the vital energy from the sun and feel invigorated.

Taking A Shower

Make your bath time a pleasurable one. While taking a shower or bathing, spend a few moments breathing consciously to bring your awareness to the present moment. This will help free your mind of any disturbing thoughts. To your surprise, you might find appropriate answers to disturbing thoughts or other questions. Be mindful as you cleanse your body.

For centuries, a great deal of emphasis has been placed on aromatherapy. As different scents and fragrances have specific effects on your mood, you may want to explore and discover what works best for you.

Mealtimes

Take time to relax and enjoy what you eat because you are what you eat. Your mood, digestion, and energy depend on the type, quality, and quantity of food you eat. Also, if you are upset or tense while eating, your body is unable to assimilate the food. Therefore, make it a point to enjoy every meal with a relaxed mind.

Driving

Sit comfortably and enjoy the driving experience. Driving is a good time to listen to your favorite music, appreciate the nature around you, or simply be aware of the present moment. Focusing your awareness towards conscious breathing while driving will further help you relax. If you are tense from thinking about your work or any other issues, simply meditate on that stressful situation to quiet your mind. For example, while driving home from work, think of the day's experiences and feel good about your hard work and pardon yourself for your shortcomings!

Breaks

Take time during your busy day to appreciate the simple yet wonderful things in your life. Practice the kind of meditation which energizes you the most. Also, practice conscious breathing for at least a few minutes to revitalize and refresh yourself. If you take a walk on your breaks or enjoy other activities, remember to breathe consciously. Nature lovers can meditate on the natural beauty they come across. If you are outside when the sun is rising or setting, take time to absorb that powerful energy by closing your eyes while facing the sun. Breathe and meditate deeply. It is very powerful and energizing!

Bedtime

This is a very important time to spend with yourself. Prior to sleeping, take few moments to rest quietly. Close your eyes and reflect on your day's work. Quickly review the things you accomplished that day. If you lived up to your expectations, simply reward yourself by thinking good about yourself. If not, do not berate yourself. Instead, meditate to learn from the day's activities. Promise to try to achieve them the next day. Remember, mistakes help us grow through experience. At the end of your meditation, remember to pray and thank God for enabling you to accomplish your goals.

Another bedtime meditation is a very powerful method to help relieve insomnia. Take a few minutes to relax quietly before sleeping. Don't invite any thoughts, but if they surface, do not suppress them. If they keep disturbing you, either meditate to find an answer or make a list of them and keep it in a visible place so you can take care of it after you get up. Most of the time worrying about uncertainties, projects, or deadlines causes insomnia, which leads to lethargy and dark circles under your eyes. Train your mind to relax, and take care of your worries after you get up in the morning.

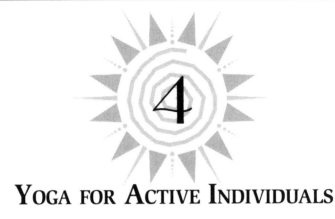

YOGA FOR ACTIVE INDIVIDUALS

(ATHLETES, DANCERS, WEIGHT LIFTERS, MARTIAL ARTISTS, & OTHERS)

"Stretching is a natural way to condition the body and prevent injuries."

Active individuals enjoy the pleasures of using their bodies and muscles in energetic and coordinated ways on a regular basis. Stretching and breathing exercises help prepare people for these activities. However, when regular stretching and body maintenance are minimized or neglected, the strain of strenuous activity on various parts of the body such as muscles, joints, ligaments, and tendons, accumulates in the body. If stretching and conditioning are not done in conjunction with strenuous activity, the accumulated stress and strain almost inevitably lead to injuries and long-term ill effects. Unfortunately by overlooking or postponing stretching, many active people have had to give up their favorite sport or activity due to some kind of permanent damage. Yoga and breathing techniques provide quick and easy ways to help stretch and strengthen the body, release accumulated stress and strain, and prevent injuries.

Kokila Patel, a registered physical therapist, relates the essential need for stretching and conditioning. "To perform well, the body needs to regularly go through its natural range of motion, keeping joints lubricated and muscles toned. For example, most lower back injuries and pain are directly related to tightness in the hip flexors, adductors, rotators, quadriceps, achilles tendon, and calf muscles due to the lack of stretching and mobilization. This neglect often leads to back sprain, herniated disc, and sciatica. It is very important for athletes, injured performers, and others to stretch properly. Stretching should be gentle, easy, and pain-free, much like Vasanthi's yoga."

Tennis players, joggers, dancers, weight lifters, body sculptors, and other athletes who incorporate yoga techniques in their activities find the benefits of yoga go beyond the effects of simple muscle stretching. These techniques help eliminate stiffness, improve coordination, and prevent injuries. Yoga also helps balance mental, emotional, and physical energy, improving concentration and endurance. Along with these benefits, yoga also helps active people release the accumulated emotional and physical tension that is stored in the body as a result of busy work schedules and daily strain.

Mythili Kumar, a prominent Bharatanatyam dancer and teacher, practices yoga to relieve ailments and improve performance. "After my first session, I rebuked myself for having waited so long. Perhaps, if I had started sooner, I would not have allowed my sinus and back problems to become chronic. The warm-up exercises that Vasanthi introduced me to led up quite easily to the more challenging yoga asanas. Vasanthi's advice to adapt the asanas to whatever was comfortable for me provided the encouragement to continue her classes. Although my dance training had made me quite flexible, two pregnancies and the irregularity of exercise and dance practice had not helped maintain all my muscles in good condition. The breathing techniques that accompanied the yoga asanas gave me a sense of well-being. Vasanthi's modified salutation to the sun posture (surya namaskara) is a great introductory stretching exercise before beginning dance practice. Also, doing yoga asanas after an intensive dance session relieves and stretches my tired muscles. I believe that many of the wrist, ankle, eye, and neck exercises taught by Vasanthi should be done by all dance students to improve their flexibility, and several yoga asanas should be adopted into a daily practice schedule to improve posture as well as concentration."

In addition to the other benefits, the gentleness of yoga stretches make them extremely suitable as preventive and healing measures recommended for various injuries athletes frequently encounter. Most of the lower back injuries and lower back pain are directly related to tightness in the waist, hips, and legs. The combination of backward and forward bending postures along with hip-stretching poses is ideal for toning and strengthening this group of muscles. Achilles tendinitis (inflammation of the large tendon at the back of the heel) can be prevented by practicing the ankle flex, mountain pose, and hip stretches. Also, stretching the quadriceps, hamstrings, and calves with forward bending and standing balancing poses is an excellent preventive method for chondromalacia (softening of the cartilage under the knee cap). Similarly, other injuries such as plantar fascitis (inflammation of the tissue in the bottom of the foot) and shin splints (inflammation of tendons on the inside of the front lower leg) may be prevented or healed with the ankle and toe stretch, standing balancing poses, and healing by visualization techniques.

Many of my students who are involved in active sports like skiing, scuba diving, and weight lifting claim that yoga has given them extra muscle conditioning and development beyond what their regular activities provide and has helped prevent the recurrence of old injuries.

Jenny Bloom, a weight trainer, practiced yoga to help heal her injuries and improve her health. "I came to Vasanthi five years ago wanting to renew a yoga practice that I had begun and left six years ago. At that time I was doing a lot of weight lifting, pushing myself very hard. During my first year with Vasanthi, I pushed myself equally hard in yoga as I continued to push myself with weights. In addition, the weight lifting was doing extreme damage to my shoulders and elbows causing bursitis and tendinitis. My doctor told me that I had to stop or severely limit my weight use. It was an injury that for many people can leave permanent damage. Vasanthi was patient with my 'overdoing-it' approach and gently coached me to slow down my practice, which led to healing. Through slowing down, focusing, and breathing, I was able to really "do" yoga, as opposed to trying to accomplish or succeed in yoga. In the last four years, my yoga practice has healed me, strengthened me, and developed muscles in me that I never had before. In the last two years I have resumed weight lifting and began running along with other activities. Not only do I not pull muscles or injure myself in these activities any more, but my yoga practice helped prepare me for other activities. With each year, I get stronger and build more stamina."

THINGS TO KNOW BEFORE BEGINNING THE PRACTICE

- Adopt the stretches that suite you. Avoid stretches that cause pain or discomfort. Remember that even stretching a little is good for you.

- For quick muscle relaxation, try to remain in the stretch for 15-30 seconds. To condition muscles, try to stay in the stretched position for 60 seconds or more.

- Remember to breathe slowly while stretching to maximize the benefits.

- For muscular and other injuries, slow, gentle stretching and visualization techniques are ideal for healing.

- For detailed descriptions of the poses, pranayama, and meditation practices, refer to the preceding chapters.

The following table summarizes the warm-up and cool-down poses and the related benefits.

WARM-UPS & COOL DOWNS	BENEFITS
Toe and back stretch	Provides immediate relief for physical tension and fatigue. Stretches the entire body.
Warrior pose	Stretches and tones the arm, neck, shoulder, bicep, hip, leg, and calf muscles.
One leg stretch	Conditions the legs and hips by providing weight lifting benefits. Tones the spine and arms.
Arm and leg stretch	Stretches and tones the neck, face, arm, spine, chest, hip and leg muscles.
Double angle stretch	Relieves muscle stiffness, relaxes, and tones the hamstrings, calves, quadriceps, hips, spine, arms, upper back, shoulder joints, and neck. Quickly relieves mental fatigue due to the rich supply of blood towards the face and head.
Deep or complete breathing	Relaxes and soothes the muscles after warm-ups.
Salutation to the sun	Stretches and tones the entire body.
Pose of the moon	Provides immediate mental relaxation. Stretches and tones the spine, hips, and sciatic nerves. Relaxes the heart muscles.
Mountain pose	Provides a great stretch for the entire body, including hamstrings, feet, ankles, spine, wrists, and palms.
Camel	Conditions and stretches the whole body.
Turtle pose	Provides immediate mental relaxation. Develops flexibility of the entire spine, hips, sciatic nerves, and neck muscles. Relaxes the heart and lungs.
Spinal twist	Strengthens the spine, arms, upper back, neck, and shoulders.
Two leg lock	Massages and tones the neck, upper back, and shoulders, and releases upper body tension. Brings mental relaxation.
Corpse relaxation	Relaxes the entire body.

WARM-UP ROUTINE

STANDING POSES

These standing poses can be practiced either before or after an activity. They are also ideal for practicing when you are outdoors or in a gym. Try to stay in the position for 15-30 seconds.

Toe and Back Stretch

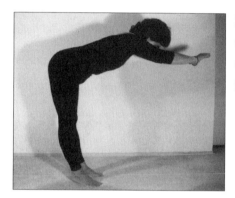

Stand on your toes. Raise both the arms to the side, then straight up. While breathing out bend forward at the waist. Breathing in come back to the standing position.

Warrior Pose

Begin by standing with feet apart. Gently turn your right foot so that it is perpendicular to the left. Raise your arms and arch backward while bending your left leg as shown. Remain in the pose for a comfortable length of time. Repeat the sequence by switching to the opposite side.

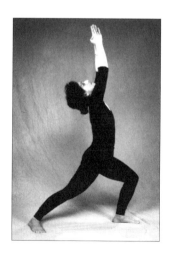

One Leg Stretch

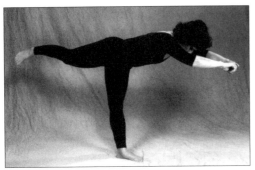

Stand straight. Balancing on one leg, lift your other leg backward and bend forward extending your arms in front of you to form a T-shape pose or as far as is comfortable. Breathe naturally. Repeat the same movements balancing on the opposite leg.

Arm and Leg Stretch

Stand straight. Bend your right leg at the knee and hold your ankle with your right hand. Lift your left arm above your shoulder. Gently lift your knee while arching your back and looking up. Breathe naturally in the position. You can also bend forward as shown in Chapter 1. Repeat these movements with the opposite leg and arm.

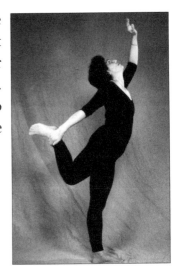

Double Angle Stretch

Stand straight with your feet a few inches or one foot apart. Clasp your hands behind your back, while straightening your arms. Move your arms slightly away from your body. Breathe in as you bend backward. Breathe out as you bend forward. Keep the arms straight while bending forward. Breathe naturally in the position. Breathing in, come up, release your hands and relax.

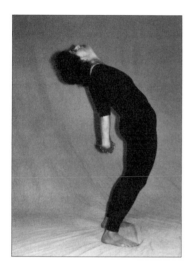 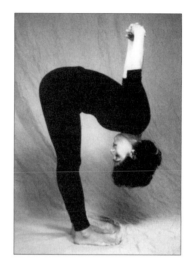

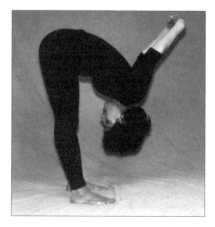

Deep or Complete Breathing

Stand with your back straight. Close your eyes. Focus your awareness on your natural breath. Gently prolong the exhalation while pulling the stomach in as much as possible. As you breathe in, let your pulled in stomach come back naturally and breathe upward while expanding the chest sideways. Breathe out from the chest to the stomach while pulling in the stomach as slowly as you can. Do this procedure gently and slowly like a smooth wave flowing up from the stomach to the chest as you breathe in and flowing down from the chest to the stomach as you breathe out. Practice this for about 15 breaths.

COOL-DOWN ROUTINE

STANDING AND SITTING POSES

This routine can be practiced either before or after an activity. They are ideal for indoor practice. Try to hold the sitting poses for 30-60 seconds.

Salutation to the Sun

When pressed for time, you may choose to practice only salutation to the sun while pausing in your favorite positions for 5-15 seconds.

Step 1. Breathe out

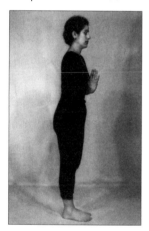

Step 2. Breathe in

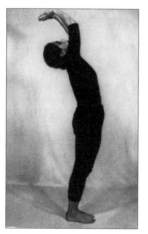

Step 3. Breathe out

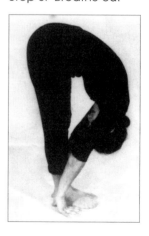

Step 4. Breathe in

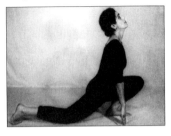

Step 5. Breathe out

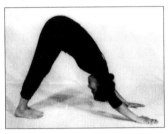

Step 6. Hold the breath

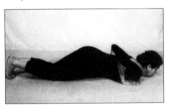

Step 7. Breathe in

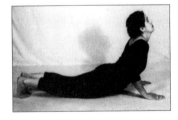

Step 8. Breathe out

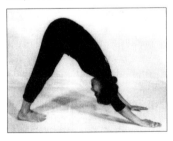

Step 9. Breathe in

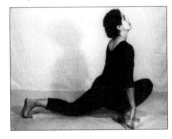

Step 10. Breathe out

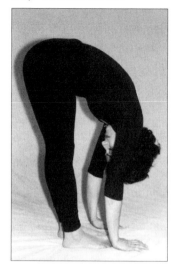

Step 11. Breathe in

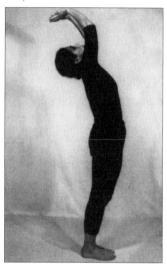

Step 12. Breathe out

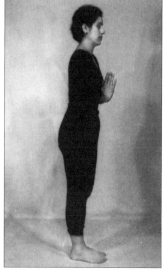

Repeat these 12-step movements moving the left leg back and forth in steps 4 and 9. This completes one round. Repeat as you wish.

Corpse Relaxation

Lie down with your arms resting slightly away from your body. With your palms facing up, relax your fingers. Rest your legs slightly apart and let your feet flop to the sides. Follow any of the corpse relaxation routines described in Chapter 2. As you are practicing, take the time to respect and appreciate your body.

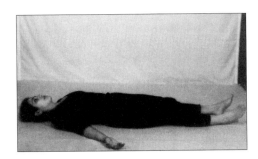

Pose of the Moon

Sit on your heels. Breathing in deeply, lift your arms straight above your head. While breathing out, pull in your stomach, lower your trunk, and rest your forehead on the floor. Close your eyes and breathe naturally. Breathing in, slowly come out of the posture and rest your arms on your knees.

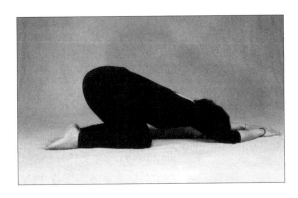

Mountain Pose

Sit on your heels with your toes bent. Bend forward so your palms rest on the floor. Raise your torso while straightening your legs and arms as shown. Lower your feet so your heels rest as close to the floor as possible. Do not use force or strain to lower your heels. Using force may strain your hamstring muscles. Bend your legs at the knee and return to the sitting position.

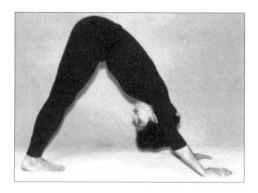

Camel

Sit on your heels with your feet flat. Allow your arms to rest at your sides.

Slowly move your arms one by one to the back, while arching your trunk backwards and slightly lowering your head. Close your eyes and maintain normal breathing. Hold the position for as long as you are comfortable. Your natural breathing becomes deeper due to the chest expansion.

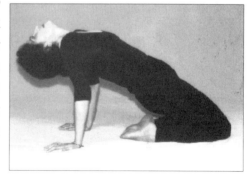

Turtle Pose

Sit on your heels. While breathing out, pull your stomach in, and rest the front part of your head on the floor as close to your knees as is comfortable. Rest your arms at your side or hold your wrists behind your back. Breathe naturally. Breathing in, come out of the posture.

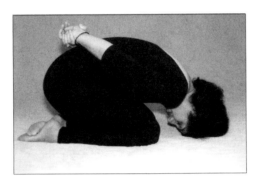

Spinal Twist

Sit with your legs extended. Cross your right leg over the left and rest your right foot or heel on the floor. Breathing out, rest your left arm over

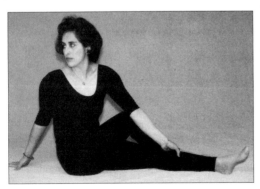

your right leg. If possible, hold your right ankle. From your waist, twist your body to the right while placing your right arm behind your back. Rest your right palm or fingers on the floor and look to the right. Your buttocks should be resting on the floor throughout this posture. Keep your body straight. Do not lean backwards or sideways. Hold the position while breathing naturally. Breathing in, release the twist and return to the sitting position. Stretch to the other side reversing the arm and leg positions.

Two Leg Lock

Lie flat on your back. Bend your legs at the knee and bring them towards your chest. Clasp your fingers around your bent legs. Breathe naturally while holding the position. Rest your head on the floor for a few moments while still in this holding position before you proceed to corpse relaxation.

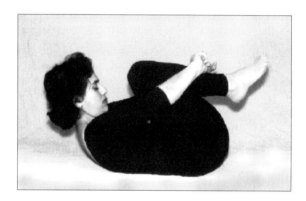

Corpse Relaxation

Lie down with your arms resting slightly away from your body. With your palms facing up, relax your fingers. Rest your legs slightly apart and let your feet flop to the sides. Breathing naturally, relax your whole body for 5-10 minutes to feel rejuvenated.

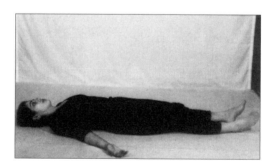

REGULAR ROUTINE

These warm-ups and poses can be practiced in addition to your other activities on a daily basis or on alternate days to tone and strengthen the body as well as to help prevent injuries.

REGULAR ROUTINE	BENEFITS
Ankle rotation and flex	Strengthens and massages the ankle, calf, and feet muscles. Provides relief for arthritic stiffness and rheumatic pain.
Butterfly	Loosens hip joints, groin, and leg muscles. Facilitates one's ability to practice the lotus or half-lotus.
Splits	Stretches the hamstring, hip and groin muscles as well as sciatic nerves.
Leg lock	Tones the neck, upper back, and shoulders, releasing upper body tension. Relaxes the sciatic nerves and hips.
Lying twist	Provides a great stretch for the hips, sciatic nerves, lower back, chest muscles, neck, and arms.
Sit-ups	Exercises the back, hips, and neck. Strengthens the abdominal muscles.
Corpse relaxation	Relaxes the entire body.
Shoulder stand	Maintains general health and helps alleviate or prevent many ailments.
Plough	Relaxes the spine and hamstrings. Relieves tiredness.
Cobra	Conditions the spine, hips, arms, and wrist joints. Complements weight lifting.
Locust	Tones the base of the spine, quadriceps, hips, and abdominal area. Provides weight lifting effects for the hips.
Bow	Stretches and massages the entire body.
Preliminary leg pull	Stretches and tones the hamstrings and spine. Relieves physical tension from the upper back.
Spinal twist	Strengthens the spine, hips, arms, upper back, neck, and shoulders.
Two leg lock	Provides benefits similar to leg lock (see above).
Corpse relaxation*	Relaxes the entire body.

* You may also practice any of the breathing techniques, such as complete breathing, bellows breath, or alternate nostril breathing before the corpse relaxation.

Ankle Rotation and Flex

Sit with your legs slightly apart and extended in front of you. Let your arms rest at your side. Rotate your feet inward several times and then outward several times, while your legs remain stationary. After rotating your feet several times in each direction, flex your feet forward and then backward. Practice this for 5-10 rounds.

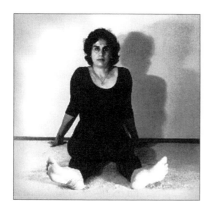 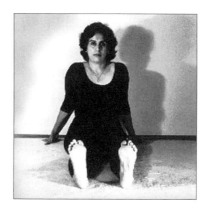

Butterfly

Sit with your legs extended and slightly apart in front of you. Bend both your legs at the knees while bringing your soles together. Interlock your fingers around your feet and pull your feet as close as is comfortable towards your body. Slowly move your knees up and down for about 30 seconds. Keeping your legs bent, try to stretch your knees towards the floor as much as possible.

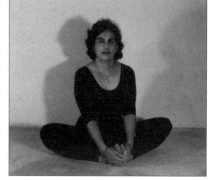

Splits

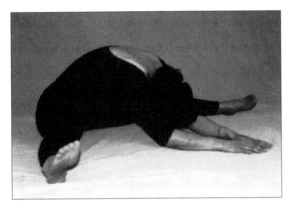

Sit with your legs apart and arms at the sides. Bend forward as you breathe out. Maintain normal breathing. Breathe in as you come out to the upright position.

Leg Lock

Lie flat on your back. Bend your left leg at the knee and bring it towards your chest. Clasp your fingers around your bent leg between your calf and

knee. As you breathe out, pull your stomach in and lift your head and upper back. Breathing in, rest your head and upper back on the floor. This is one round. Repeat 3-5 times. Practice this sequence with your right leg.

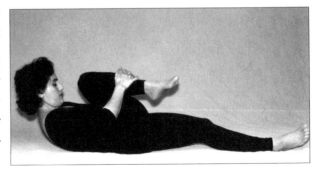

Lying Twist

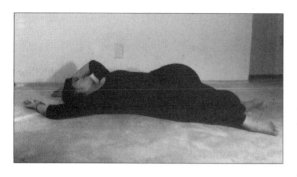

Lie flat on your back. Bend your legs at the knees, keeping your feet flat on the floor. Cross your right leg over your left leg and drop your legs to the left. With your legs on your left side, stretch your arms above your head and to the right. Also, turn your head to the right. Hold this position with your eyes closed for as long as is comfortable while breathing naturally. Come out of the position. Then cross your left leg over your right leg as shown and repeat this procedure in the opposite direction.

Sit-Ups

Lie flat with your legs bent at the knees, arms resting at your side. Breathing out, lift your upper body and arms towards your knees as much as possible. Breathing in, rest your upper body on the floor. Repeat 10-15 times.

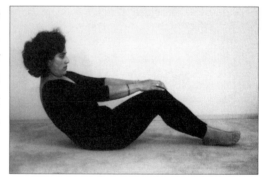

Corpse Relaxation

Lie down with your arms resting slightly away from your body. With your palms facing up, relax your fingers. Rest your legs slightly apart and let your feet flop to the sides. Follow any of the corpse relaxation routines described in Chapter 2.

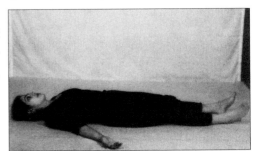

Shoulder Stand

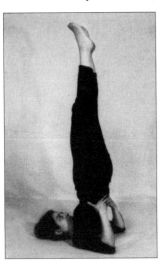

Lie flat on your back, with your arms at your sides, palms pressing against the floor. Breathing out, slowly lift your trunk and legs while tightening your abdominal and leg muscles. Breathe normally in this position. Hold your lower back to support your trunk. Straighten the trunk and legs as much as possible while lowering your hands for further support. Practice rectal contractions to accelerate the benefits. Slowly lower your trunk, rest your palms on the floor and lower your legs to return to the resting position. Be sure to relax completely before repeating this posture or attempting any other posture.

Plough

Lie flat on your back, with your arms at your sides, palms pressing against the floor. Breathing out, slowly lift your trunk and legs, while tightening your abdominal and leg muscles. You may hold your trunk for additional support. Lower your legs until they are parallel to the floor. 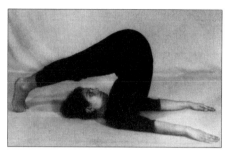 Breathe naturally in the position. Listen to your body and proceed. Be sure to pull your stomach in while breathing out as you lower your legs further until your toes touch the floor. At this point, you may remove your hands from your back and rest them on the floor. Stay as long as you are comfortable. Slowly come out of the position while resting your arms on the floor. Relax completely before repeating this posture or attempting another posture.

Cobra

Lie on your stomach, arms resting at your side and chin resting on the floor. Move your palms in front of or just below your shoulders. As you breathe in, straighten your arms and lift your trunk off the floor. Stretch as much as you can with the lower 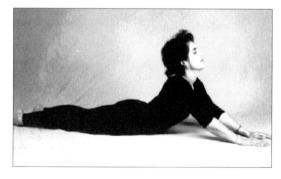 part of your stomach on the floor. Try to look up. Breathe naturally. Hold this position for a comfortable length of time. Breathing out, lower your trunk and head, resting your cheek on the floor.

Locust

Lie on your stomach, arms resting at your side and chin resting on the floor. Make a tight fist and hold it below or beside your hip joints. Breathing naturally, lift your legs while pressing your arms against the floor. Stay in this position for 5-10 seconds. Do not strain in order to stay longer in this asana, as it could cause tension to the heart. Come out of the position slowly and rest your cheek on the floor with arms at your sides.

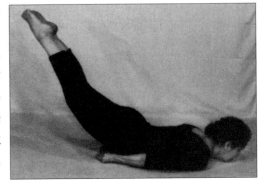

Bow

Lie on your stomach, arms resting by your side and chin on the floor. With your legs bent, hold your ankles and lift your legs and upper body. Stay in this position for 10-15 seconds. Come out of the position and rest your cheek on the floor.

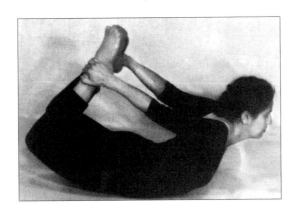

Preliminary Leg Pull

Sit with your legs extended and your hands resting on your legs. Breathing in deeply lift your arms above your head. Breathing out, pulling in your stomach, bend forward and slide your arms as far as possible. Hold your legs comfortably. Breathe naturally while holding the position. Breathing in deeply come back to a seated position.

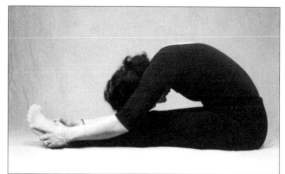

Spinal Twist

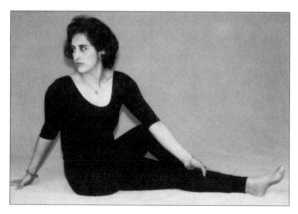

Sit with your legs extended. Cross your right leg over the left and rest your right foot or heel on the floor. Breathing out, rest your left arm over your right leg. From your waist, twist your body to the right while placing your right arm behind your back. Rest your right palm or fingers on the floor and look to the right. Your buttocks should be resting on the floor throughout this posture. Keep your body straight. Do not lean backwards or sideways. Hold the position while breathing naturally. Breathing in, release the twist and return to the sitting position. Stretch to the other side reversing the arm and leg positions.

Two Leg Lock

Lie flat on your back. Bend your legs at the knee and bring them towards your chest. Clasp your fingers around your bent legs between your calf and knee. As you breathe out, pull your stomach in and lift your head

and upper back. Hold the position for 10-15 seconds breathing naturally. Breathing in, rest your head and upper back on the floor. Keeping your legs bent, hold this position for a few seconds before proceeding with the corpse relaxation.

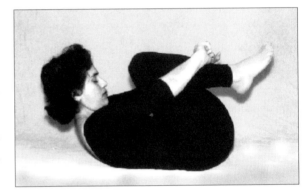

Corpse Relaxation

Lie down with your arms resting slightly away from your body. With your palms facing up, relax your fingers. Rest your legs slightly apart and let your feet flop to the sides. Practice slow and deep breathing for 2-5 minutes. While breathing in, experience the relaxation throughout the body. Breathing out, release any accumulated physical, emotional, and mental tension.

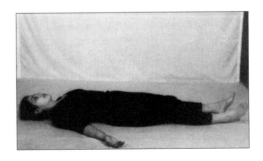

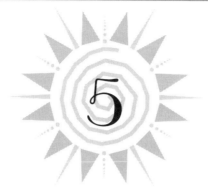

YOGA IN THE WORKPLACE

"Your performance and productivity depend upon the balance between your body, mind, and breath."

With technological advancement in the business world, greater and greater demands are placed on us. As these demands increase, more stress accumulates in our lives irrespective of whether we work in a high-tech business, school, retail store, restaurant, garden, home, or in any other occupation. Our inability to reduce our stress levels and take care of our needs affects our daily performance, which over the years adversely affects our lives.

The routines described in this chapter are designed to enable busy people to incorporate stress-relief, relaxation, and meditation techniques into their daily work schedules. These techniques are also highly effective for relieving the strain and fatigue of constant sitting, standing, repetitive movements, and other work-related symptoms. You can practice these techniques while at work, while traveling, or whenever there is a need to feel invigorated. When practiced regularly, they can help relieve stress, improve concentration, and boost self-confidence.

George Joseph, a software engineer, eased his back pain with these techniques. "I have been practicing yoga with Vasanthi since 1993. Despite having limited use of my right leg due to polio, I am able to utilize yoga to strengthen my back muscles. I no longer have any lower back pain in spite of my disability and my busy working schedule."

Jatinder Singh, a restaurant manager, found relief from insomnia by practicing a combination of forward bending, backward bending, and spinal twist postures, followed by deep breathing, breath counting, and vipasana meditation. "As a restaurant manager, I experienced extreme stress due to employee turnover and long, unpredictable hours. Under pressure from upper management, I was restless and sometimes slept for only a few hours for several weeks. After trying sleeping pills for many weeks, I called Vasanthi for suggestions and started practicing stress management and meditation techniques from her audio and video tapes. Within a short time, I was able to sleep well and to my surprise, relieve my allergies. I now practice yoga everyday!"

Sandra Needs, a legal administrative coordinator, says, "I originally started yoga because of the benefits promised from improved breathing techniques. I had suffered from a chronic sinus infection and had also developed asthma as an adult. Yogic breathing techniques did indeed help both of those conditions, but an unexpected benefit was the reduction in upper back pain and muscle tightness associated with working at a computer and using a computer mouse. My shoulders are much more relaxed and if I do feel tightness coming on, I now have specific yoga techniques to relax my back and shoulders."

THINGS TO KNOW BEFORE BEGINNING THE PRACTICE

- Adopt a routine that suits your needs.
- You may still practice your regular yoga and meditation in addition to these routines.
- For detailed descriptions of the poses, pranayama, and meditation practices, refer to the preceding chapters.

The routines in this chapter include:

- *ONE MINUTE BREATHING ENERGIZERS*

- *QUICK RELAXATION MOVEMENTS*

- *INSTANT TENSION RELIEVERS*

- *RELAXATION FOR THE MIND*

ONE MINUTE BREATHING ENERGIZERS

To relax before you start your day, practice all or any of the following meditation and breathing techniques.

Early Morning Meditation

The moment you are awake, take time to observe your breath flow. If you have deadlines, complicated work, presentations, or are just thinking of the day's challenges, it can cause an emotional imbalance which immediately affects your breath. Close your eyes and meditate on your breath flow. Visualize the positive outcome of your work and take pride in what you do. This will not only improve your self-esteem, but will enable you to deal with situations with alertness and ease. Your positive thoughts will calm your mind and ease your breath flow. When your breath flow is steady, practice deep breathing a few times.

This technique can be practiced throughout the day to replenish your energy and reduce stress or anxiety.

Alternate Nostril Breathing

Rest your index and middle fingers of your right hand between the eyebrows. Close your right nostril with your thumb. Breathe in comfortably through your left nostril. Close the left nostril with your ring finger. Open the right nostril and breathe out. Now, breathe in through the right nostril, close that nostril, and breathe out through your left nostril. This is one round. Repeat 3-5 rounds.

This technique develops will power, relieves emotional stress, and balances energy. When practiced before public presentations, it is also a very effective method to alleviate nervousness by calming and balancing the nervous system.

Complete Breathing

Sit comfortably with your back straight. Close your eyes. Focus your awareness on your natural breath. Gently prolong the exhalation while pulling the stomach in as much as possible. As you breathe in, let your pulled in stomach come back naturally and breathe upward while expanding the chest sideways. Make sure not to expand your stomach more than normal. This expansion can restrict the flow of air to the upper chest. Breathe out from the chest to the stomach while pulling in the stomach as slowly as you can. Practice this procedure gently and slowly like a smooth wave flowing up from the stomach to the chest as you breathe in and flowing down from the chest to the stomach as you breathe out. Practice for about 15 breaths.

This technique quickly relaxes the entire system and helps alleviate nervousness, anxiety, anger, and fatigue. It also boosts self-confidence before public speaking.

QUICK RELAXATION MOVEMENTS

For quick relaxation and stress relief, you can practice all or any of these techniques in a seated position.

Neck Movements

Sit with your back straight and move your head up as you breathe in. Then lower your head as you breathe out. Now tilt you head to your left shoulder and then to your right shoulder. Rotate your head clockwise and counterclockwise several times.

These movements relieve stiffness and tension from the neck and help alleviate mental fatigue.

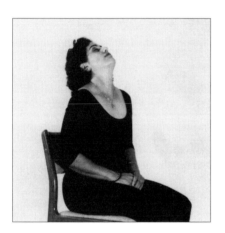
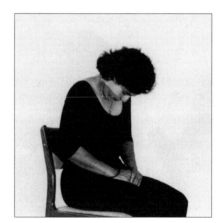
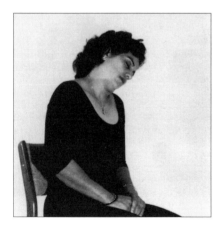
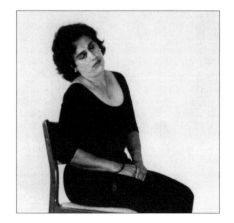

Hand and Wrist Joint Stretch

Sit with your back straight and extend your arms straight in front of you at the shoulder level. Make a tight fist with fingers over your thumbs. Hold it for 5-10 seconds. Release and stretch your fingers as far out as possible. Practice several times and repeat when you need it.

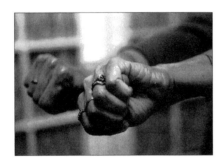 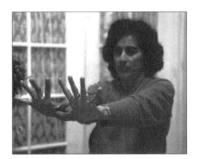

With your arms held straight, move your palms up and hold it for 5-10 seconds. Then move your palms down, pivoting at the wrists. Repeat as needed. Make a fist with your fingers over your thumbs. Slowly rotate your wrists inward and then outward several times.

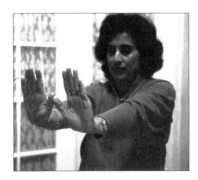 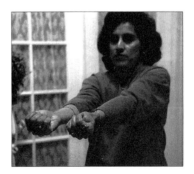

These techniques relax and tone the wrist joints, arms, and fingers. They also help treat carpal tunnel syndrome, arthritis, and tendinitis.

Shoulder and Arm Stretch

While seated with your back straight, interlock your fingers, raise your arms over your head, and stretch out as you arch backwards. Stay in this position for a few seconds. Return to the upright position. Repeat 3-5 times.

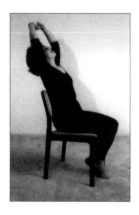 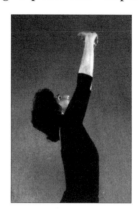

This technique relieves fatigue and relaxes the muscles of the upper back, neck, shoulders, and arms.

Leg and Feet Stretch

Sit with your back straight. Stretch your feet while lifting your legs as high as is comfortable. Rotate your feet inward and outward several times.

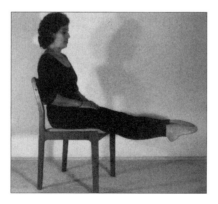

This technique relaxes the feet and calms the mind due to its effect on the pressure points.

Spine Stretch and Twist

Sit with your back straight. Breathing in, stretch your arms in front of you and then up over your head as much as possible. Breathing out, slowly lower your arms towards the floor, bending from the hips and allowing your head to hang loose. Hold this position while breathing naturally. Stay in this position as long as you are comfortable. Stretching the arms further helps relax the neck, shoulder area, and spine. Breathe in deeply as you come up. From there, cross your right leg over your left and twist your body towards your right as shown below. Repeat this on the other side by crossing your left leg over your right.

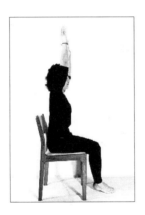
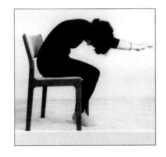
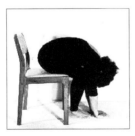
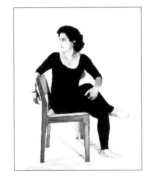

This technique is an overall relaxer and rejuvenator. The forward bending position increases circulation to the head, relieving mental fatigue. The spinal twist helps release energy from the base of the spine.

Eye Exercises

The following eye exercises are effective methods to improve your eyesight and help relieve various discomforts. I started wearing glasses for shortsightedness at the age of seven. My eyesight got progressively worse for years until I started practicing these eye exercises. Within 6 months, my eyesight improved, and I was able to get rid of my glasses. These exercises also helped me relieve my dry eyes which I had for many years.

Practice 1

Sit with your back straight and raise your eyebrows as you look up. While still looking up, close your eyes and hold the stretch for a few seconds. Release the stretch and open your eyes to complete one round. Repeat 3-5 times.

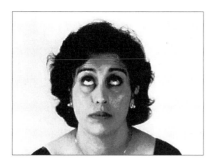 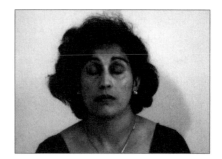

This practice stretches and relaxes the optical nerves and helps reduce outer-eye wrinkles.

Practice 2

Look up and pause for a few seconds. Then gradually rotate your eyes clockwise (as shown on the next page), pausing between movements. Close your eyes and relax for a few seconds between rotations. Practice this 2-3 times. Repeat the same movements counter-clockwise. You may gradually increase this practice to 5 rotations.

This exercise relaxes tired eyes and helps improve eyesight.

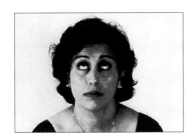

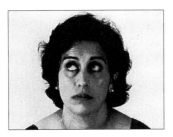

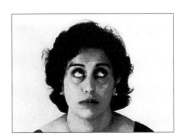

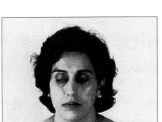

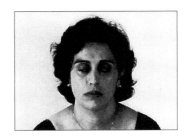

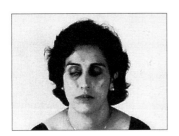

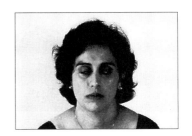

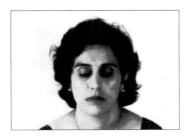

Practice 3

Bring your fingertip between your eyebrows and focus on the tip of your finger. Slowly move your finger down to the tip of your nose, keeping your concentration on your fingertip. Try not to blink while moving your finger. However, there is a tendency to blink when your eyes naturally release tears. Repeat 3-5 times.

Next, close your eyes and place your palms over your closed eyelids and hold for a few seconds or for as long as you wish. This is known as palming.

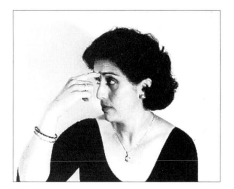 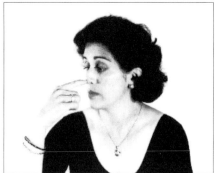

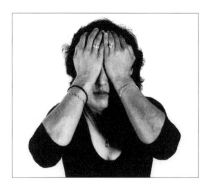

This practice lubricates dry eyes, soothes tired eyes, and relaxes the optic nerves.

INSTANT TENSION RELIEVERS

Toe Stretch

Stand on your toes. Raise both the arms to the side and then straight up. While breathing out, bend forward. Breathe naturally. Breathing in, come back to the standing position.

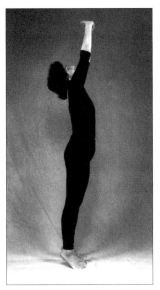
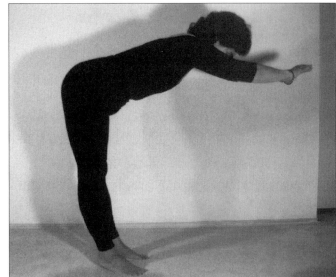

Feet and Palm

Standing straight, breathe in and stretch your arms up as you arch your back. As you breathe out, bend down as much as possible. Breathe naturally and focus on parts of the body where you experience stretch and blood circulation.

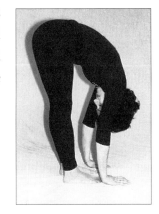

Double Angle

Stand straight with your feet about one foot apart. Clasp your hands behind your back and straighten your arms. Move your arms slightly away from your body. Breathe in as you bend backward. Breathe out as you bend forward. Keep your arms straight while bending forward. Breathe naturally in this position for 15-30 seconds. Breathing in, come up and release your hands as you relax.

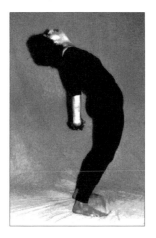 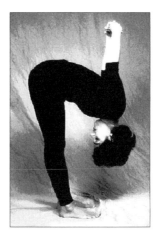

These techniques are excellent for relieving physical and mental fatigue. Forward-bending poses enhance memory and alertness, relax the eyes, and bring a glow to the face.

RELAXATION FOR THE MIND

Breath Meditation

Practice deep breathing and feel your breath flow in and out through your nostrils. As you breathe in, feel the prana (vital energy) flow into your body. As you breathe out, feel the tension leaving your body.

This technique calms your nerves when you experience frustration. It also quickly refreshes you and helps relieve mental fatigue. You may find this technique very useful prior to an important meeting or before making an important phone call. You can also adopt this technique to energize yourself when taking a walk or performing your exercise routine.

Room Enhancement

Make a special effort to arrange your workplace so that it relaxes you. For example, you may decorate the walls with pictures of your favorite vacation spots, nature scenes, or other esthetically pleasing colors and accessories. You may place photographs of your loved ones on your desk. Keep in mind that your environment plays a vital role in creating a positive mood.

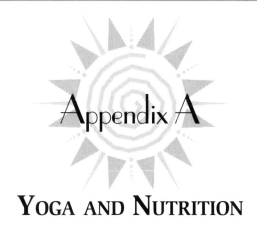

YOGA AND NUTRITION

Along with air, sun, water, and sleep, food is one of our primary sources of vital energy. Nutritious eating habits can complement our attitude, health, and energy level. In order to maintain our health or lose weight, we have to be conscious of what we eat. It is also essential to remember that a diet that is appropriate for one person, may not always be appropriate for another. For example, while one person's appetite may be satisfied with one bowl of food, another individual may need two bowls. Therefore, there is no need to struggle to lose weight by worrying about the quantity of food you eat. Losing weight is not necessarily accomplished by eating less. Rather, a healthy diet consists of increasing the intake of nutritious foods, while decreasing the intake of unhealthy foods.

Our frame of mind or attitude towards food is also very important. Reminding ourselves to relax while eating, makes our meal times valuable and enjoyable. If we eat happily, we are less likely to put on weight because our body is able to assimilate the food better through a calm and activated digestion process.

HINTS FOR A HEALTHY DIET

For a healthy diet, try to include some or all of these suggestions.

- Include a large portion of grains (carbohydrates), such as rice, pasta, wheat, and oats.
- Eat plenty of fruits and vegetables, such as banana, apple, pear, broccoli, and green leafy vegetables which are rich in vitamins and minerals.
- Include an ample portion of dairy products as well as beans and legumes (garbanzo, lentils, red and black eyed beans, and others).
- Try to eat fresh or frozen foods in place of canned foods as much as possible. Fresh foods contain more vital energy than preserved foods.
- Never skip breakfast.
- Drink plenty of water.

HINTS FOR WEIGHT LOSS

To promote weight loss, try to follow the Hints for a Healthy Diet along with some or all of the following suggestions.

- Reduce your intake of salt by avoiding salty foods because excess salt causes water retention, leading to extra body weight.
- Decrease the amount of fatty foods in your diet and increase your intake of fiber.
- Drink at least 5-6 cups (8 oz.) of water a day to cleanse your system.

Provided below is a guideline you could use to modify your diet if you are striving to lose weight. The quantities specified are only approximate. Use your judgement in planning your meals. For example, to lose weight,

IF YOUR NORMAL DIET INCLUDES SOME OF THE FOLLOWING:	MODIFY YOUR DIET TO THE FOLLOWING:
2-3 slices of bread	1- 11/2 slices
1 cup of cooked rice	1/2 cup of cooked rice
2-3 chapatis or tortillas	1- 11/2 chapati or tortilla
1/4 cup of cooked lentils or beans	1/2 cup of cooked lentils or beans
1/2 cup of cooked or steamed vegetables	1 cup of vegetables
1/2 bowl of salad	1 full bowl of salad
2 servings of fruit	3 servings of fruit
Low fat milk	Nonfat milk
1 cup of buttermilk or yogurt	1 cup of low fat or nonfat yogurt
2 cups of juice	2 cups of sugar-free juice
2-3 cookies or 2 servings of any dessert	1 cookie or 1/2 serving of any dessert

Practice your favorite warm-ups and postures with steady breathing regularly. When practicing pranayama techniques, remember to select deep breathing, bellows breath, and alternate nostril breathing so you can emphasize exhalation. Good exhalation helps eliminate toxins, and stimulate the digestive process, and encourages deep inhalation. Good inhalation helps convert fat cells into energy, enabling you to be active.

In addition, walk or exercise regularly, making it a pleasurable experience. When pressed for time, make the most of your environment. For example, climb stairs instead of using elevators. Increase your walk by parking your car in a farther spot when you go shopping, or increase your activities at home when you are house bound.

Appendix B

SUGGESTED ROUTINES FOR GENERAL HEALTH

&

SPECIFIC AILMENTS

The routines listed below provide an easy way to practice yoga in order to heal or prevent specific ailments. They can also be practiced as short routines for general health and relaxation when you are pressed for time. For additional benefits, you may also incorporate these suggested yoga techniques in your regular practice routines.

Abdominal ailments (menstrual cramps, acidity, diabetes): Leg lock, churning the mill, pose of the moon, turtle, camel or cobra, preliminary leg pull, spinal twist, slow deep breathing (sitting, standing, or lying), gentle bellows breath, and healing by visualization meditation.

Abdominal strengthening and reducing: Sit-ups, boat, cobra, locust, bow, preliminary leg pull, camel or fish, turtle pose, spinal twist, deep breathing, bellows breath, and abdominal lift.

Acne: Salutation to the sun, shoulder stand, plough, preliminary head stand, cobra, bowing pose, complete breathing, and alternate nostril breathing.

Alertness: Bowing pose, mountain pose, preliminary head stand, bellows breath, bee sounding breath, and breath counting meditation. Conscious breathing alone helps!

Anger: Vipasana meditation, complete breathing, alternate nostril breathing, and conscious breathing.

Anxiety: Pose of the moon or bowing pose, cobra, preliminary leg pull, spinal twist, complete breathing, alternate nostril breathing, and vipasana and chanting meditation.

Arthritis: Stretching conditions the muscles and improves circulation, so practice any given routine daily.

Back pain: Churning the mill, leg lock (one and two leg), lying twist, pose of the moon, turtle, cat, plough or mountain pose, cobra (easy step), preliminary leg pull, and spinal twist.

Balancing energy: Bowing pose, cat, mountain pose or preliminary headstand, shoulder stand, plough, cobra, preliminary leg pull, spinal twist, alternate nostril breathing, and vipasana meditation.

Blood pressure:
> **High**: Any of the warm-ups, except salutation to the sun. Corpse relaxation, cat, pose of the moon, cobra, preliminary leg pull, alternate leg pull, and spinal twist. Simple breathing, alternate nostril breathing, counting and chanting breath meditation (without breath retention), and vipasana meditation.
> **Low**: Salutation to the sun, corpse relaxation, pose of the moon, preliminary head stand or mountain pose, cat, shoulder stand, plough, cobra, preliminary leg pull, alternate leg pull, and spinal twist. Simple breathing, alternate nostril breathing, counting and chanting breath meditation (with breath retention), and vipasana meditation.

Cancer:

> **Breast**: Lying twist, cobra, bow, pose of the moon (easy variation), camel, cat, and spinal twist. Incorporate healing by visualization meditation separately or in the postures along with slow deep breathing.

> **Colon**: Pose of the moon, plough, cobra, plane, preliminary leg pull, spinal twist, bellows breath, and abdominal lift.

> **Prostate**: Rectal contraction, shoulder stand, plough or preliminary head stand, plane, and bowing pose. Practice healing by visualization separately or in the postures along with slow deep breathing.

> **Lung**: Cobra (easy step), pose of the moon, camel stretch A, bowing pose, deep breathing, panting breath, lion breath, alternate nostril breathing, and healing by visualization meditation.

Carpal tunnel syndrome: Hand and wrist stretch, double angle, camel, mountain pose, cobra and bowing pose.

Cold:

> **Immediate relief**: Deep breathing, alternate nostril breathing, and bellows breath.

> **Prevention**: Salutation to the sun, mountain pose, fish or camel, bowing pose, cobra, (locust and bow stretch can be included in the advance practice), pose of the moon, spinal twist, complete breathing, lion breath, and alternate nostril breathing.

Concentration: Bowing pose, preliminary head stand, turtle pose, alternate nostril breathing, and counting breath meditation.

Depression: Bowing pose, preliminary headstand, cobra, pose of the moon, bellows breath, alternate nostril breathing, vipasana meditation, chanting, and yoga nidra meditation.

Double chin: Warrior pose, salutation to the sun, camel, cat, cobra or fish, bowing pose, and spinal twist.

Drug addiction: Cooling breath, alternate nostril breathing, bellows breath, complete breathing, vipasana and yoga nidra meditation. Morning (sunrise) or evening (sunset) walk is recommended.

Energizing: Bowing pose, cat, preliminary head stand, cobra or camel, preliminary leg pull, turtle, complete breathing, bellows breath, alternate nostril breathing, and corpse relaxation.

Eyes:
> **Dryness & itching**: Practice eye exercises 1 and 3.
> **Vision improvement**: Practice eye exercises 1, 2, and 3. Include head down and backward bending poses, such as mountain pose, pre liminary head stand, shoulder stand, plough, cobra, bowing pose, spinal twist, and others. (Open your eyes and stretch your eyes for a few moments while in the backward bending poses.)
> To reduce or eliminate eye glasses or contact lenses, try to wear glasses with slightly lesser power than you actually need. (Consult your optometrist.) Remove glasses during yoga practice. Include carrots and salads in your diet.

Face:
> **Face lift treatment**: Warrior pose, arm and leg stretch, cobra, bow, cat, camel or fish, bowing pose, spinal twist, and eye exercises.
> **Wrinkles**: Eye exercises and backward/forward bending poses.

Fatigue:
> **Mental fatigue**: Bellows breath, deep breathing, and any head down poses.
> **Physical fatigue**: Leg lock, lying twist, double angle, feet and palm stretch, salutation to the sun, corpse relaxation, preliminary head stand, cobra, turtle, spinal twist, and corpse relaxation.

Headache: Pose of the moon, shoulder stand, plough, cobra, bowing pose, alternate nostril breathing, rhythmic breathing, and vipasana meditation on stressful situations in order to overcome worries and uncertainties.

Hamstring: Standing balancing poses, mountain pose, plough, preliminary leg pull, alternate leg pull, and splits.

Hair loss: Feet and palm stretch, shoulder stand, plough, preliminary head stand, bowing pose, turtle pose, and pose of the moon. Be sure to include fruits and vegetables in your diet.

Healing injuries: Healing by visualization meditation and gentle stretches.

Heart: Standing balancing poses, salutation to the sun, turtle, pose of the moon, cobra, locust, bow, shoulder stand, plough, preliminary leg pull, psychic union pose, alternate leg pull, lying and sitting twists, and corpse relaxation. Complete breathing, alternate nostril breathing, rhythmic breathing, and vipasana meditation.

> **Blocked arteries**: Practice the techniques recommended for the heart, replacing the shoulder stand and plough with the mountain pose. Healing by visualization meditation separately and in the postures, breathing techniques without breath retention, and corpse relaxation.

Hemorrhoids: Rectal contraction as often as possible. Shoulder stand, plough, locust, plane, and preliminary head stand (with rectal contraction). Increase fiber foods in your diet.

Hot flash: Cooling breath and alternate nostril breathing.

Insomnia: Leg lock, lying twist, cobra, preliminary leg pull, spinal twist, alternate nostril breathing, and rhythmic breathing. Meditate before bedtime to balance your mental disturbances or set them aside until you wake up.

Lung ailments:

 Allergy: Salutation to the sun, corpse relaxation, shoulder stand, plough, fish, turtle pose, cobra, plane, bow, pose of the moon, spinal twist, complete breathing, alternate nostril breathing, bellows breath, panting breath, and lion breath.

 Asthma and Emphysema: Leg lock, lying twist, cobra, preliminary leg pull, camel or fish, bowing pose, and spinal twist. Complete breathing, bellows breath, panting breath, and alternate nostril breathing. (Maintain slow and steady breathing while you practice.)

Memory: Feet and palm stretch, bowing pose, pose of the moon, preliminary head stand, shoulder stand, plough, fish, turtle, bee sounding breath, and counting breath meditation.

Menopause: Adopt any practice routine from Appendix C.

Neck (neck pain and whiplash): Leg lock, lying twist, neck movements, half plough or mountain pose, cat, cobra (easy step) or plane stretch, preliminary leg pull, alternate leg pull, and spinal twist.

Nervousness: Alternate nostril breathing with breath retention, complete breathing, and bellows breath.

Osteoporosis: Adopt any practice routine from Appendix C and extend the duration of each pose.

Pimples: Salutation to the sun, shoulder stand, plough, cobra, bowing pose, preliminary head stand, complete breathing, alternate nostril breathing, and cooling breath. Minimize the fat content in your diet.

Sinus congestion: Bowing pose, chin lock A, and/or alternate nostril breathing with chin lock.

Smoking: Refer to routines suggested for drug addiction.

Snoring: Lying twist, two leg lock, cobra, bowing pose, turtle, spinal twist, bellows breath, panting breath, lion breath, bee sounding breath, complete breathing, and om chanting.

Sore throat: Energy renewing breathing, lion breath, bee sounding breath, complete breathing, and healing by visualization meditation.

Spiritual uplifting: Regular practice of postures, breathing, vipasana meditation, and mantra chanting.

Stamina: Salutation to the sun, corpse relaxation, bellows breath, panting breath, and complete breathing. Adopt a well-balanced diet.

Stress: Leg lock, lying twist, plough or mountain pose, cobra, preliminary leg pull, turtle pose, spinal twist, simple breathing, complete breathing, and alternate nostril breathing.

Thyroid: Salutation to the sun, corpse relaxation, shoulder stand, plough, fish, psychic union pose, camel, turtle, cobra, locust, bow, preliminary leg pull, turtle pose, lying twist, and spinal twist. Alternate nostril breathing, lion breath, om chanting, and corpse relaxation. Incorporate healing by visualization meditation in the practice.

Varicose veins: Shoulder stand, plough, plane, locust, preliminary leg pull, mountain pose or preliminary head stand, and standing balancing poses.

Vocal chords: Fish or camel, turtle, panting breath, lion breath, bee sounding breath, and om chanting.

Youthfulness: Regular practice of hatha yoga.

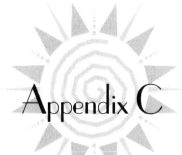

Appendix C

PRACTICE ROUTINES

GENERAL ROUTINES

ROUTINE 1

Ankle rotation
Butterfly
Splits
Leg lock
Lying twist
Neck movements
Triangle stretch
Half lotus tree pose
Double angle
Corpse relaxation
Pose of the moon
Mountain pose
Camel (*A, and either B or C*)
Shoulder stand
Plough
Cobra
Preliminary leg pull
Spinal twist
Two leg lock
Complete breathing
Bellows breath
Alternate nostril breathing
Corpse relaxation

ROUTINE 2

Churning the mill
Hip stretch
Cobra
Plane
Bow
Preliminary leg pull
Cat
Preliminary head stand
Bowing pose
Spinal twist
Abdominal lift
Energy renewing breathing
Alternate nostril breathing
Om chanting
Corpse relaxation

ROUTINE 3

Salutation to the sun (*2-3 rounds*)
Corpse relaxation
Shoulder stand
Plough
Fish
Psychic union pose
Alternate leg pull
Spinal twist
Two leg lock
Vipasana meditation
Yoga nidra meditation and rest

ROUTINE 4

Salutation to the sun
Corpse relaxation
Shoulder stand
Plough
Fish
Psychic union pose
Camel
Pose of the moon
Cobra
Locust
Bow
Preliminary leg pull
Preliminary head stand
Cat
Turtle pose
Alternate leg pull
Spinal twist
Yoga nidra meditation

ROUTINE 5

Leg lock
Lying twist
Sit-ups to boat stretch
Corpse relaxation
Shoulder stand
Plough
Cobra
Turtle pose
Preliminary leg pull
Spinal twist
Bellows breath
Alternate nostril breathing
Corpse relaxation

QUICK ROUTINES

ROUTINE 1

Salutation to the sun *(1-3 rounds)*
Corpse relaxation
Bellows breath

ROUTINE 2

Mountain pose *or*
Preliminary headstand
Bowing pose
Cobra
Preliminary leg pull
Spinal twist
Alternate nostril breathing
Corpse relaxation

ROUTINE 3

Feet and palm stretch
Arm and leg stretch
Toe and back stretch
Warrior pose or triangle stretch
Double angle stretch
Double breath *(standing)*
Complete breathing *(standing)*
Corpse relaxation *(optional)*

ROUTINE 4

Pose of the moon
Cat
Cobra
Locust or plane
Bowing or turtle pose
Lying twist
Two leg lock
Any 2 breathing techniques
Vipasana meditation
Corpse relaxation

ROUTINE 5

Toe and back stretch
Warrior pose
Double angle stretch
Abdominal lift
Salutation to the sun *(2 rounds)*
Corpse relaxation

ROUTINE 6

Bowing pose
Preliminary headstand
Cat
Pose of the moon
Turtle pose
Spinal twist

VASANTHA YOGA
HEALTH & FITNESS PRODUCTS

Vasantha Yoga offers a wide range of video products for general health and fitness. These tapes provide a guided yoga practice for people of all age groups and physical conditions. The most recent release includes a compact disc and an audiotape titled 'Meditation for All Walks of Life'.

These products are sold in the United States as well as in other countries. They offer very clear and simple demonstrations of Vasanthi's unique and gifted style of teaching. These techniques complement the yoga practice described in this book. A convenient order form is provided at the end of this section.

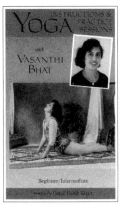

YOGA INSTRUCTIONS & PRACTICE SESSIONS
BEGINNER/INTERMEDIATE
$ 39.95

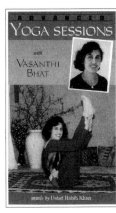

ADVANCED YOGA SESSIONS
LEVEL I
$ 29.95

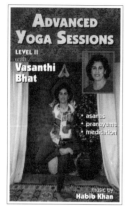

ADVANCED YOGA SESSIONS
LEVEL II
$ 29.95

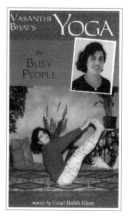

YOGA FOR BUSY PEOPLE
$ 29.95

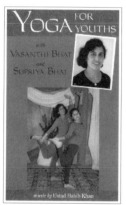

YOGA FOR YOUTHS
$ 29.95

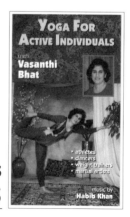

YOGA FOR ACTIVE INDIVIDUALS
$ 29.95

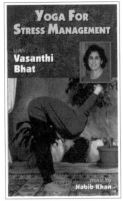

YOGA FOR STRESS MANAGEMENT
$ 24.95

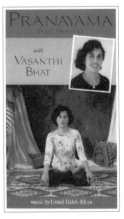

PRANAYAMA LEVEL I
$ 19.95

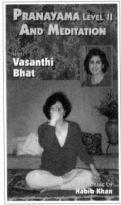

PRANAYAMA LEVEL II & MEDITATION
$ 24.95

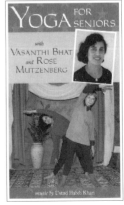

YOGA FOR SENIORS
$ 24.95

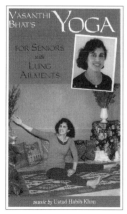

Yoga for Seniors with Lung Ailments
$ 19.95

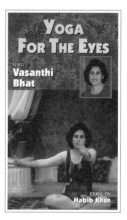

Yoga for the Eyes
$ 19.95

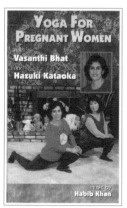

Yoga for Pregnant Women
$ 19.95

Meditation For all Walks of Life

Compact Disc
$12.95

Audio Tape
$ 6.95

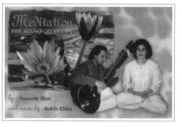

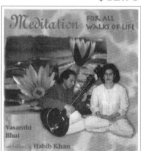

Cut along dotted line

VASANTHA YOGA ORDER FORM

SPECIAL

25% DISCOUNT

on any videotape, audiotape, or compact disc order with the purchase of this book.

VIDEO TAPE	UNIT PRICE	QTY	AMOUNT
YOGA INSTRUCTIONS & PRACTICE SESSIONS	$39.95	X _____	= _____
ADVANCED YOGA SESSIONS LEVEL I	$29.95	X _____	= _____
ADVANCED YOGA SESSIONS LEVEL II	$29.95	X _____	= _____
YOGA FOR BUSY PEOPLE	$29.95	X _____	= _____
YOGA FOR YOUTHS	$29.95	X _____	= _____
YOGA FOR ACTIVE INDIVIDUALS	$29.95	X _____	= _____
YOGA FOR STRESS MANAGEMENT	$24.95	X _____	= _____
PRANAYAMA LEVEL I	$19.95	X _____	= _____
PRANAYAMA LEVEL II & MEDITATION	$24.95	X _____	= _____
YOGA FOR SENIORS	$24.95	X _____	= _____
YOGA FOR SENIORS WITH LUNG AILMENTS	$19.95	X _____	= _____
YOGA FOR THE EYES	$19.95	X _____	= _____
YOGA FOR PREGNANT WOMEN	$19.95	X _____	= _____

AUDIO TAPE

MEDITATION FOR ALL WALKS OF LIFE	$6.95	X _____	= _____

COMPACT DISC

MEDITATION FOR ALL WALKS OF LIFE	$12.95	X _____	= _____

PAPERBACK

THE POWER OF CONSCIOUS BREATHING IN HATHA YOGA	$19.95	X _____	= _____

Sub Total _____

Shipping & Handling $4 per item _____

(Add $2 for every additional item) _____

California residents add 8.25% Sales Tax _____

Total _____

Make check payable to 'Vasanthi Bhat' and mail to:

VASANTHA YOGA
1196 Lynbrook Way, San Jose CA 95129
For information, call 408.257.8418 or e-mail: vasanthib@aol.com

Cut along dotted line

VASANTHA YOGA ORDER FORM

SPECIAL

25% DISCOUNT

on any videotape, audiotape, or compact disc order with the purchase of this book.

VIDEO TAPE	UNIT PRICE	QTY	AMOUNT
YOGA INSTRUCTIONS & PRACTICE SESSIONS	$39.95	X _____	= _____
ADVANCED YOGA SESSIONS LEVEL I	$29.95	X _____	= _____
ADVANCED YOGA SESSIONS LEVEL II	$29.95	X _____	= _____
YOGA FOR BUSY PEOPLE	$29.95	X _____	= _____
YOGA FOR YOUTHS	$29.95	X _____	= _____
YOGA FOR ACTIVE INDIVIDUALS	$29.95	X _____	= _____
YOGA FOR STRESS MANAGEMENT	$24.95	X _____	= _____
PRANAYAMA LEVEL I	$19.95	X _____	= _____
PRANAYAMA LEVEL II & MEDITATION	$24.95	X _____	= _____
YOGA FOR SENIORS	$24.95	X _____	= _____
YOGA FOR SENIORS WITH LUNG AILMENTS	$19.95	X _____	= _____
YOGA FOR THE EYES	$19.95	X _____	= _____
YOGA FOR PREGNANT WOMEN	$19.95	X _____	= _____

AUDIO TAPE

MEDITATION FOR ALL WALKS OF LIFE	$6.95	X _____	= _____

COMPACT DISC

MEDITATION FOR ALL WALKS OF LIFE	$12.95	X _____	= _____

PAPERBACK

THE POWER OF CONSCIOUS BREATHING IN HATHA YOGA	$19.95	X _____	= _____

Sub Total _____

Shipping & Handling $4 per item _____

(Add $2 for every additional item) _____

California residents add 8.25% Sales Tax _____

Total _____

Make check payable to 'Vasanthi Bhat' and mail to:

VASANTHA YOGA
1196 Lynbrook Way, San Jose CA 95129
For information, call 408.257.8418 or e-mail: vasanthib@aol.com

.

VASANTHA YOGA ORDER FORM

SPECIAL

25% DISCOUNT
on any videotape, audiotape, or compact disc order with the purchase of this book.

VIDEO TAPE

	UNIT PRICE	QTY	AMOUNT
YOGA INSTRUCTIONS & PRACTICE SESSIONS	$39.95	X _____	= _____
ADVANCED YOGA SESSIONS LEVEL I	$29.95	X _____	= _____
ADVANCED YOGA SESSIONS LEVEL II	$29.95	X _____	= _____
YOGA FOR BUSY PEOPLE	$29.95	X _____	= _____
YOGA FOR YOUTHS	$29.95	X _____	= _____
YOGA FOR ACTIVE INDIVIDUALS	$29.95	X _____	= _____
YOGA FOR STRESS MANAGEMENT	$24.95	X _____	= _____
PRANAYAMA LEVEL I	$19.95	X _____	= _____
PRANAYAMA LEVEL II & MEDITATION	$24.95	X _____	= _____
YOGA FOR SENIORS	$24.95	X _____	= _____
YOGA FOR SENIORS WITH LUNG AILMENTS	$19.95	X _____	= _____
YOGA FOR THE EYES	$19.95	X _____	= _____
YOGA FOR PREGNANT WOMEN	$19.95	X _____	= _____

AUDIO TAPE

MEDITATION FOR ALL WALKS OF LIFE	$6.95	X _____	= _____

COMPACT DISC

MEDITATION FOR ALL WALKS OF LIFE	$12.95	X _____	= _____

PAPERBACK

THE POWER OF CONSCIOUS BREATHING IN HATHA YOGA	$19.95	X _____	= _____

Sub Total _____

Shipping & Handling $4 per item _____

(Add $2 for every additional item) _____

California residents add 8.25% Sales Tax _____

Total _____

Make check payable to 'Vasanthi Bhat' and mail to:

VASANTHA YOGA
1196 Lynbrook Way, San Jose CA 95129
For information, call 408.257.8418 or e-mail: vasanthib@aol.com

NOTES

NOTES

NOTES

NOTES

NOTES

Notes